D1558693

Physiology of the Eye

Physiology of the Eye

An Introduction to the Vegetative Functions

Second Edition

Irving Fatt, Ph.D.
Professor Emeritus
School of Optometry
University of California, Berkeley

Barry A. Weissman, O.D., Ph.D.
Professor of Ophthalmology
Jules Stein Eye Institute and Department of Ophthalmology
School of Medicine
University of California, Los Angeles

Butterworth–Heinemann
Boston London Oxford Singapore Sydney Toronto Wellington

Library of Congress Cataloging-in-Publication Data
Fatt, Irving.
    Physiology of the eye : an introduction to the vegetative
functions / Irving Fatt, Barry A. Weissman. — 2nd ed.
       p.   cm.
    Includes bibliographical references and index.
    ISBN 0-7506-9085-2 (sewn)
    1. Eye—Physiology.   I. Weissman, Barry A.   II. Title.
    [DNLM: 1. Eye—physiology.   WW 103 F254p]
    QP475.F28   1992
    612.8'4—dc20
    DNLM/DLC
    for Library of Congress   92-12311
                                                          CIP

British Library Cataloguing-in-Publication Data.
A catalogue record for this book is available from the British Library.

Butterworth–Heinemann
80 Montvale Avenue
Stoneham, MA 02180

10   9   8   7   6   5   4   3   2   1

Printed in the United States of America

Contents

Preface to the Second Edition

The objectives of this text remain the same as those stated in the Preface to the first edition. The book was written as a text for optometry students but will be useful to all who need a summary of the vegetative processes carried out in the human eye. The definition of *vegetative* remains the same; it describes those processes operating in the eye to maintain it as a viable organ in the face of forces that are trying to break down the organ's tissues. As in the first edition, discussion of the eye as a processor of visual information is not included.

The organization of the book remains the same as in the first edition with the exception of an extra chapter on the cornea. Since the writing of the first edition, about 15 years ago, the increased use of contact lenses has brought about a need for more detailed knowledge by fitters of contact lenses, both optometrists and ophthalmologists, of corneal physiology. However, no introductory text can provide all of the details now known about the cornea's response to a contact lens, nor can it provide the most current knowledge. The reader is urged to maintain a close watch of the optometric and ophthalmic literature in the contact lens field.

The sequence of topics in the first edition of this text was chosen to correspond to the sequence in Hugh Davson's *The Eye*, Volume 1, published by Academic Press in 1969 so that students could use both as texts in their studies. In 1984 Dr. Davson published a new edition of his work (*The Eye*, Volumes 1a and 1b, 3rd Edition, Academic Press). This more modern version of *The Eye* is recommended as a supplement to this text in a course on vegetative physiology of the eye.

Acknowledgments

As is true for most books, the authors could not have completed this one without the assistance and encouragement of many. We both extend our appreciation to our families for their support.

Many colleagues assisted in the preparatation of various portions of this text, giving guidance and encouragement. We wish to thank Gordon L. Fain, Joseph Horowitz, David A. Lee, Hillel Lewis, Bartley J. Mondino, Roger L. Novak, Thomas H. Pettit, and Bradley R. Straatsma, all of UCLA. Special thanks for providing Figures 6.1 to 6.5 are due to Jan P.G. Bergmanson of the University of Houston. We also thank Mrs. Carolyn Buck Reynolds for the redrawn anatomical details of the eye given in Figures 1.2, 1.3, 1.5, and 1.6 and for the artwork of Figures 10.1, 10.7, and 10.8.

Any errors, oversights, or omissions are regretted; these are clearly our own.

1

Review of Ocular Anatomy

Although there are philosophical objections to a teleological approach to the study of the eye, that is, treating the eye as a device designed to carry out certain desired processes, much of the vegetative physiology of the eye is best grasped through such an approach. Our modern technological society gives us certain intuitive feelings for mechanisms and how they carry out their required functions. If we believe that each part of the eye has its own special function and carries out this function in at least a satisfactory, if not always optimal, fashion, then we must understand the elements and interactions of ocular anatomy for an understanding of ocular function.

Many anatomical elements of the eye are best described and understood in connection with their function. For this reason, only gross anatomy is described in this chapter. Most of the detailed anatomy, as necessary, will be described in later chapters when physiological function is discussed. For those who are interested there are several detailed texts concerned solely with ocular anatomy, histology, and physiology.

The eye is an organ in which patterns of light are brought into focus on the retina, and the ensuing chemical reaction leads to an electrical signal propagated in the optic nerve. Although the analogy to a manmade camera cannot be pursued too far, there are enough similarities to make such an analogy useful.

A cross-section of the eye (Figure 1.1) displays the following elements: the two-lens optical system of *cornea* and *crystalline lens;* a variable diaphragm, the *iris;* a shutter, the *lids;* a light-tight box, the *sclera;* and a photosensitive surface, the *retina.* The extraocular muscles serve to point the eye in the desired direction, within the limits imposed by the bony socket of the orbit.

The physical limitations of body tissue and fluid as the building materials of the eye dictate the manner in which the eye is constructed. To obtain both a fast and a wide-angle rotation, the eye must be a sphere in a well-lubricated socket. Maximum physical protection is achieved by extending the orbit over almost the entire globe. The optical system of the human eye is not focused by changing the distance between the lens and the photosensitive surface, as is done in both some cameras and lower animals such as certain fish. (Walls [1942] discusses the interesting

1

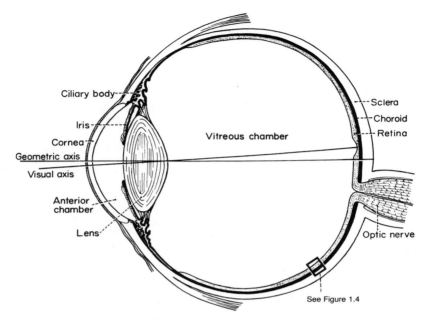

Figure 1.1 Sagittal section through a human eyeball. The area of the retina surrounded by a box at lower right is shown in detail in Figure 1.4. (From Davson H [ed.] [1969]: The Eye, Vol. 1. New York, Academic Press.)

focusing adaptations of vertebrate eyes in detail.) Instead, focusing is achieved by changing the refractive power of the crystalline lens through action of the ciliary muscle. To prevent stray light from confusing the image on the retina, the entire optical system must be set in a light-tight chamber. The cornea is the transparent outermost optical element, but it is set into the sclera, which, together with its highly pigmented *choroid* lining, acts as the light-tight covering. (As will be discussed later, both the cornea and sclera are composed of similar protein fibers, the only difference being in the organization of these fibers.)

GROSS ANATOMY

The mammalian eye is a sphere, slightly flattened in the anteroposterior direction. The *geometrical axis* passes through the center of the cornea and the lens and intersects the sclera at the posterior pole. The *visual axis* is not coincident with the geometrical axis, however, passing through both the nodal point of the optical system and the most sensitive portion of the retina, the fovea (see Figure 1.1). If the geometrical axis is treated as analogous to the earth's north–south axis, then the equator is a circle centered on this axis. A meridional section is then analogous to a section along the lines of longitude. A sagittal section runs in an anteroposterior direction along the vertical meridian.

The sagittal diameter of the human eye, along the geometrical axis, is about 24 mm. Other diameters are much less well defined. The vertical diameter, a vertical line connecting opposite points on the equator and intersecting the geometrical axis, is about 23 mm in humans. The analogous horizontal or transverse diameter is about 23.4 mm (Davson 1969).

The posterior half of the human eyeball is almost spherical. The sclera of the anterior half is flattened. On this flattened sphere is the cornea. Maurice (1969) likens this situation to a purse string drawn and tightened at the junction of the cornea and sclera. This junction is called the *limbus*. There is actually a depression, known as the *corneal sulcus* or *external scleral sulcus*, at this junction, but this depression is filled with soft conjunctival tissue.

INTERNAL ANATOMY

The globe may be divided into three tissue layers, the fibrous tunic, the uveal tunic, and the retina.

Sclera and Cornea

The outer case of the eye is known as the *fibrous tunic*. It serves, when inflated by the internal fluid pressure, to give shape to the eye and to protect the delicate internal structures. The outermost layer of the tunic is *Tenon's capsule*, a thin dense connective tissue layer overlying the *episclera*. The episclera can be distinguished from the sclera itself by being more loosely woven and rich in blood vessels. Below the episclera is the *sclera*. The outer layers of the sclera are joined to a sheath, the *dura mater*, which is a continuation of the membrane covering the brain.

The protein fibers are arranged into ribbons or *lamellae* in the sclera, and these in turn are interwoven to give strength and inelasticity. The lamellae have two main directions: in the anterior portion they run parallel to the limbus, but at the equator the lamellae begin to run meridionally and then proceed to cross each other at right angles in the posterior half of the globe. The thickness of the sclera varies at different points on the eye. In the human eye the sclera is about 0.6 to 0.8 mm at the limbus, thinning to 0.4 to 0.5 mm at the equator and thickening again to 1.0 mm in the posterior pole; under the tendons of the extraocular muscles the sclera may be as thin as 0.3 mm (Hogan et al. 1971).

The sclera is pierced by numerous nerves and blood vessels, but neither travel along its interior. The blood vessels observed on a "blood-shot" eye are in the outer, loose conjunctiva and episcleral tissue covering the sclera. A few living but nonreproducing cells, known as *fibroblasts*, are found in the sclera. *Pigment cells* similar to those found in the choroid are also present in large numbers in the sclera, particularly on the inner surface.

When the scleral lamellae cross the limbus into the cornea they undergo a change in fiber organization. This change, which is described in detail in Chapter 6, leads to the transparency of the cornea contrasted to the opacity of the sclera.

The cornea is a thin, convex—concave lens bathed on the posterior surface by liquid *aqueous humor* and separated from the air on the anterior surface by a microscopically thin layer of tears. The *in vivo* thickness of the human cornea in its central region is about 0.52 mm, thickening to about 0.67 mm at the limbus. The central radius of corneal curvature is about 7.8 mm (with some variation), and topographically it flattens peripherally to become more elliptical than spherical toward the limbus; its chord diameter is about 11.7 mm (Hogan et al. 1971).

Corneal structure is complex when studied in detail but can be divided into five recognizable layers in humans. From anterior to posterior, these layers are the *epithelium* with its *basement membrane, Bowman's layer, stroma, Descemet's membrane,* and the *endothelium.* The epithelium and endothelium are purely cellular layers, about 50 μm and 5 μm thick, respectively. The stroma is the major structural element, amounting to some 90% of the total thickness, but it has only 2% cells by volume, the *keratocytes,* the remainder being water, collagen fibers, and a jelly-like ground substance. Bowman's membrane is a modification of the stroma, and Descemet's membrane is the basement membrane of the endothelial cell layer; these are both quite thin.

Corneoscleral Junction

The limbus is the junction where the five-layer cornea joins the sclera. The corneal epithelium and Bowman's membrane undergo modification at the limbus to become the conjunctiva. The interface between stroma and sclera is, in cross-section, concave toward the stroma, giving the appearance, as Walls (1942) says, that the cornea is set into the sclera like a watch crystal in its bezel. In cross-section (Figure 1.2), it can be seen that immediately posterior to the junction is a vessel, the *canal of Schlemm,* that makes a complete circle around the cornea. The *trabecular meshwork* separates this canal from the aqueous humor. The canal of Schlemm has outlet conduits, the *aqueous veins,* which penetrate the sclera and join veins running on the anterior surface of the globe. The function of this system of vessels is to drain the aqueous humor from the chamber between the cornea and the lens, as will be described in detail in Chapter 2.

Uvea

The *uveal tunic* is a layer of tissue covering the inside surface of the sclera. The posterior segment of the uvea is the *choroid,* a thin, deeply pigmented layer consisting mostly of blood vessels with a connective tissue meshwork binding them into a membrane. Toward the front of the eye, the uvea thickens to form the *ciliary body.* In a cross-section taken meridionally, the ciliary body has a triangular shape with two long sides and one short side. The short side forms part of one wall of the anterior chamber. One long side lies along the sclera, and the other faces the vitreous chamber (see Figure 1.1).

The ciliary body is in large part a smooth muscle, the *ciliary muscle,* whose function is to change the shape of the crystalline lens during the process of

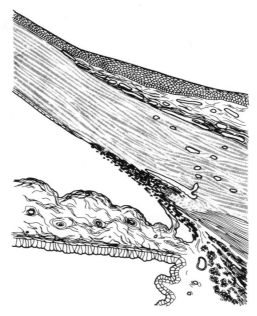

Figure 1.2 Details of the corneal–scleral junction. The corneal epithelium, seen on top of the cornea, progresses to the right to become the scleral epithelium. The horizontal member is the iris, which joins the sclera to form an angle. The lumen of Schlemm's canal is shown at the root of this angle. (Adapted from Hogan MJ, Alvarado JA, Weddell JE, [1971]: Histology of the Human Eye. Philadelphia, W.B. Saunders Co. With permission.)

focusing. When the ciliary muscle contracts, the elastic tension in the suspensory fibers of the lens is relaxed. The lens is thus allowed to assume a more rounded or convex shape and thereby bring the images of near objects into focus on the retinal surface.

The surface of the ciliary body is covered with two layers of epithelial cells below which is a capillary bed: the *unpigmented epithelium,* which is continuous with the neurosensory retina, and underlying *pigmented epithelium,* which is continuous with the retinal pigment epithelium. Invagination of the optic cup during development causes these two layers of cells to become apposed, apex to apex, and there are tight junctions, probably representing the blood–aqueous barrier, between these cells. Intercellular borders may be offset between the two layers, and interdigitation of cells may occur. The basal luminal membrane of the nonpigmented cells is highly infolded.

The junction between the retina and the ciliary body is serrated and therefore called the *ora serrata.* Anterior to the ora serrata, and extending for about two-thirds of the length of the ciliary body, is the relatively smooth *pars plana* or *orbiculus ciliaris.* The remaining anterior one-third of the ciliary body is the strongly folded *pars plicata* or *corona ciliaris.* The peaks of these folds are the *ciliary processes,* and between them are the *ciliary valleys.* The convoluted nature of the corona ciliaris serves to increase its surface area, an important factor in the production of aqueous humor.

The thin contractile tissue called the *iris* (Figure 1.3) projects from the anterior base of the triangular ciliary body. The posterior surface of the iris is covered by a heavily pigmented layer of epithelial cells; this layer makes the iris light-tight and contributes to eye coloration. Anterior to this *posterior pigmented epithelium* is a layer of specialized epithelial cells, with muscular basal portions, which make up the *dilator iridis* muscle. Both epithelial layers are supported

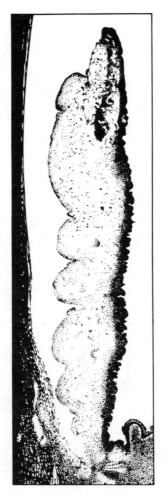

Figure 1.3 Section through the iris. The posterior layer of the epithelial cells is shown as a dark band on the right. The edge of the pupil is at the top; the iris root is at the bottom. (Adapted from Hogan MJ, Alvarado JA, Weddell JE [1971]: Histololgy of the Human Eye. Philadelphia, W.B. Saunders Co. With permission.)

anteriorly by the iris *stroma,* which is the main connective tissue body of the iris and contains the iris *sphincter muscle.* In blue-eyed individuals, the stroma has very little pigment, and the blue color is an optical effect of the posterior pigmented epithelium being seen through the translucent stroma. The stroma is moderately pigmented in green eyes and heavily pigmented in brown eyes. The most anterior layer is called the *anterior border layer,* which differs from the stroma by having less collagen and more cells, especially melanocytes.

At the border of the *pupil,* the round central hole in the iris, the *dilator iridis* becomes connected with a strong muscular structure, the *sphincter iridis* or *sphincter pupillae.* The dilator and sphincter muscles work in antagonism to adjust the size of the pupil in response to impulses arising in the nervous system. The main antagonist of the muscle closing the iris is simply the tissue elasticity and the inflated iris blood vessels.

The stromal layer of the iris is a delicate and pliable tissue. Microscopic examination shows empty spaces leading to gross openings in the anterior border layer. These openings are known as the *iris crypts.* It appears then that the iris stroma is bathed by aqueous humor.

The iris has little rigidity and a portion of it rests on the lens. The effect of contact between the lens and iris is to push forward the pupillary part of the iris, thereby forming a truncated cone.

Retina

The inner layer of the shell of the eye is the *retina.* This is composed of ten layers, the innermost nine of which make up the *neural retina* and the outermost of which is the non-neural *retinal pigment epithelium.* This tissue is anatomically-ically characterized by a high degree of regularity in its structural elements. When described in detail, the structure of the retina appears backward (Figure 1.4). The photoreceptors, composed of both *rods* and *cones,* are farthest from the vitreous–retinal interface and are in contact with the single-layered pigmented epithelium, which is in turn laid down on the choroid. Internal to the layer of rods and cones is a meshwork of neural tissue made up of the embedded nerve cell bodies and their interconnected fibers. The innermost layer of the retina is made up of only nerve fibers and an overlying vascular arborization. The combination of blood and melanin pigment in both retina and underlying choroid gives a characteristic pink-orange color to the ocular fundus. A freshly dissected and dark-adapted retina is also pink due to rhodopsin in the photoreceptors, but after exposure to light the adaptive process will turn the retina colorless. This appears to be reversible as long as the retinal pigment epithelium is intact and functioning.

The retina is not uniform over its entire surface. In the human eye there is a circular area about 5.0 mm in diameter lying slightly temporal and inferior to the geometrical posterior pole; this area is called the *macula.* The photoreceptors are more slender and densely packed in this area. In the very center of the macula the retina thins considerably, allowing even greater exposure of the photoreceptor layer directly to incoming light.

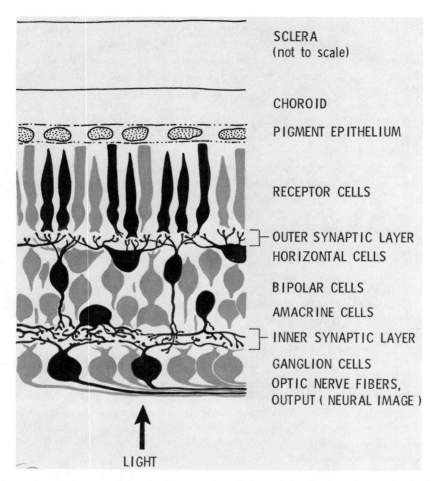

SCLERA
(not to scale)

CHOROID

PIGMENT EPITHELIUM

RECEPTOR CELLS

OUTER SYNAPTIC LAYER
HORIZONTAL CELLS

BIPOLAR CELLS

AMACRINE CELLS

INNER SYNAPTIC LAYER

GANGLION CELLS
OPTIC NERVE FIBERS,
OUTPUT (NEURAL IMAGE)

LIGHT

Figure 1.4 Structure of the vertebrate retina. A few cell bodies have been selectively stained by the Golgi method to emphasize the details of their structure. (From "The Control of Sensitivity in the Retina" by F.S. Werblin. Copyright 1973 by Scientific American, Inc., all rights reserved.)

The nerve fibers on the surface of the retina converge into an oval area located about 3 mm nasal to and just a little below the posterior pole; this is called the *optic disk, papilla,* or *nerve head.* The nerve fibers converging on this disk form bundles or fascicles of fibers, and these fibers turn at right angles to penetrate the sclera through a sieve-like structure called the *lamina cribrosa.*

A more detailed description of the structure of the neural retina is beyond the scope of this work (and more appropriate in a volume on the visual processes operating in the eye), but some of the biophysical and biochemical properties of the retina will be discussed in Chapter 9.

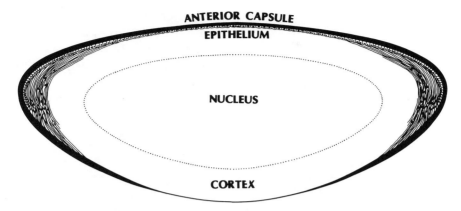

Figure 1.5 Cross-section of the adult human lens.

Crystalline Lens

The two refractive elements of the eye, the cornea and the crystalline lens, together form a compound lens. For brevity, in the remainder of this text the term *crystalline lens* will be shortened to *lens*.

The healthy lens is a transparent, biconvex, semisolid body. In newborn humans, it has a slightly yellowish tinge that becomes darker with age. The geometrical centers of the anterior and posterior surfaces of the lens are called the *anterior* and *posterior poles,* respectively. The rounded-off junction of these surfaces is called the *equator.*

The lens is composed of a mass of transparent cells, most of which are very elongated and therefore called *lens fibers.* Enclosing the lens is an elastic membrane called the *lens capsule.*

The anterior surface of the lens (under the lens capsule) is covered with a cuboidal cell layer known as the *lens epithelium.* These are the only nucleated, dividing cells in the lens. As these cells divide, they are pushed gradually toward the equator (Figure 1.5), where they line up in encircling rows. As the cells elongate, they are first pushed into the bow region and then later they extend both forward under the epithelium and backward until the ends meet at the poles to form structures called *sutures.* As these cells continue to elongate and become lens fibers, they gradually lose their nuclei, mitochondria, and ribosomes, becoming continuously less metabolically active. Each row of cells, organized into an equatorial circle, becomes a layer of fibers laid down on the previous layer. In this manner the lens continually grows concentrically, compressing the older fibers as they become more deeply buried. The zone of newer fibers is called the *cortex,* whereas the inner zone of harder, older fibers is called the *nucleus.*

The suspensory mechanism used to change the shape of the lens in the process of focusing is known as the *suspensory ligament* or *zonule of Zinn,* abbreviated as the *zonule.* The zonule may be divided into anterior and posterior leaves; the fibers of the anterior leaf originate at the anterior surface of the lens near the equator and run to the folds on the surface of the ciliary body facing the posterior chamber (Figure 1.6), whereas the posterior leaf runs from the posterior surface of the lens, also near the equator, to a zone on the orbiculus ciliaris about 1.5 mm in front of the ora serrata.

Vitreous Body

The *vitreous body* is a transparent, colorless mass of gel-like material that fills the vitreous chamber (see Chambers of the Eye, following) to form the major portion of the interior of the eye. The vitreous gel may break down with aging to become a liquid; this is common in humans beyond middle age. Although there have been reports describing a membrane surrounding the vitreous, none is convincing.

The vitreous body has a roughly spherical shape when free of the eye. This structure is solid because the interior is a network of collagen fibers with the space between these fibers filled with a glycosaminoglycan gel. The vitreous body has a

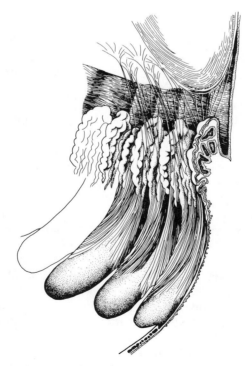

Figure 1.6 Details of the suspension of the lens (*top right*) by fibers originating at the ciliary body. (Adapted from Hogan MJ, Alvaredo JA, Weddell JE [1971]: Histology of the Human Eye. Philadelphia, W.B. Saunders Co. With permission.)

saucer-shaped depression, the *patellar fossa,* at its anterior pole where it fits to the posterior surface of the lens, leaving a potential space.

The fibers of the vitreous body attach to the surface of the posterior and vitreous chambers at three zones. Anteriorly, the vitreous adheres to the epithelium of the orbiculus ciliaris in a zone near the ora serrata; this firm anchorage has been called the *vitreous base.* Another anterior attachment lies around the rim of the patellar fossa and is called the *ligamentum hyaloideocapsulare of Wieger.* Posteriorly the vitreous has a circular attachment in the macular area and another about the optic disk. From within this latter attachment zone a tubular opening through the fiber network of the vitreous extends to the center of the patellar fossa. This opening is a remnant of the space occupied by the hyaloid artery during fetal life. There are no blood vessels or nerves in the normal vitreous body after birth, and there is only a very small number of living cells. Detachments of the vitreous may occur as part of the aging process as well.

Chambers of the Eye

The entire spherical internal volume of the eye is filled with either tissue, liquid, or a gel-like liquid. For descriptive purposes the three liquid- or gel-filled spaces are given special names.

Just behind the cornea, and in front of the iris, is the *anterior chamber.* Small parts of the sclera, lens, and ciliary body, the posterior corneal surface, and the entire anterior surface of the iris form the boundaries of this chamber. The anterior chamber is filled with a transparent, colorless liquid, the *aqueous humor,* which is produced by the epithelial cells of the ciliary body. Aqueous humor provides nutrition to much of the inner eye and serves as a flowing stream into which metabolic waste may be disposed. This aqueous humor leaves the eye, for the most part, through the canal of Schlemm, which is located in the corneoscleral junction.

The *posterior chamber,* also filled with aqueous humor, is the space bounded by the posterior surface of the iris, the equatorial portion of the lens, the anterior surface of the vitreous body, and the inner surface of the ciliary body. The *canal of Hannover* or *circumlental space* is the space bounded by the two leaves of the zonule and equatorial zone of the lens. And finally, there is some anatomical evidence for a space between the posterior leaf of the zonule and the surface of the vitreous body, known as the *retrozonular space* or *canal of Petit.*

The *vitreous chamber* is directly behind the lens and the zonule and is filled with a gel, the vitreous body.

Blood Vessels in the Eye

The *ophthalmic artery* supplies all of the arteries of the eyeball. Similarly, all of the major veins of the eye usually discharge into the ophthalmic vein. Arteries and veins divide into the retinal and ciliary systems before entering the eye. These systems remain separate within the globe (Figure 1.7).

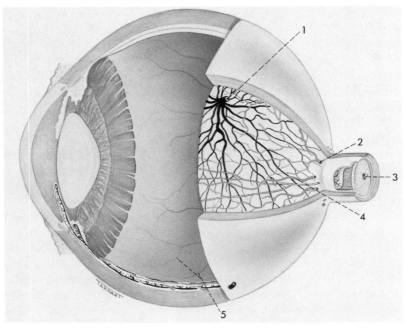

Figure 1.7   Section through a human eye showing the distribution of blood vessels. The dark vessels are veins; the gray vessels are arteries. The anatomical feature shown as a double line at the center of the eyeball is the ciliary nerve.

The *central retinal artery,* arising from the ophthalmic artery at the apex of the bony orbit, is the arterial source of the retinal system. The central retinal artery enters the nerve sheath 7 to 15 mm behind the globe and runs along the axis of the nerve bundle. Branches from this artery supply the cells of the nerve sheath and the nerve itself. The artery enters the eye in the middle of the optic disk.

The retinal veins run alongside the retinal arteries. They join into a *central retinal vein* that leaves the eye alongside the central retinal artery in the axial portion of the optic nerve. The central retinal vein finally joins with the *ophthalmic vein,* which is the major venous channel within the orbit and which drains, via the spheroidal fissure, into the *cavernous sinus.*

The ciliary arterial system supplies all parts of the eye except the retina. The short *posterior ciliary arteries* penetrate the sclera along an eccentric circle around the optic nerve. They then enter the choroid and divide into fine branches to form the *choriocapillaris.* Some of the posterior ciliary arteries send branches toward the intraocular portion of the optic nerve to form the *intrascleral arterial circle of Haller* or *Zinn.* These arteries supplement the blood supply from the retinal arteries. In some eyes the intrascleral arterial circle sends branches, known as *cilioretinal arteries,* into the retina where they appear on the disk close to its temporal border and then run to the macular area.

The two *long posterior ciliary arteries* pierce the sclera forward from the entrance of the short posterior ciliary arteries, pass forward between the sclera and the choroid, and enter the ciliary body partway along its length. Near the root of the iris, but still within the ciliary body, the two arteries bifurcate and the branches join end-to-end to form a major arterial circle in the anterior uvea, called the *major arterial circle of the iris.* Additional arteries contributing to this circle are known as the *anterior ciliary arteries,* which arise from the muscular branches of the ophthalmic artery and reach the eye via the four rectus muscles. These arteries run forward in the episcleral tissue from the insertion of the muscles, pierce the sclera 3 to 4 mm behind the limbus, and then connect with the major circle. The branches of this major circle provide blood to the ciliary muscles and the iris. Fine episcleral branches of the artery join with the conjunctival vessels to form the limbal network or *marginal plexus.*

The venous channels of the eye are especially important because, in addition to leading the circulating blood out of the eye, they have as their function the drainage of the aqueous humor from the anterior chamber. The *anterior ciliary veins* collect venous blood from the anterior scleral and episcleral plexuses as well as from the ciliary body. Most of the venous blood is carried away from the iris and ciliary body, together with all choroid venous blood, by the *vortex veins.* These veins pierce the sclera obliquely near the equator and connect with the larger orbital veins.

Nonvisual Nerves of the Eyeball

The muscles of the iris and ciliary body, parts of the vascular system, and the corneal surface are supplied with sensory and autonomic innervation.

The sensory innervation for the eye arises from the *nasociliary nerve,* a prominent branch of the fifth cranial (trigeminal) nerve. The ophthalmic division of the fifth nerve is joined to the eyeball and lids by sympathetic fibers that have their origin in the *superior cervical ganglia.* The cells in these ganglia are in turn connected with nerve fibers that have come up via the cervical sympathetic trunk from the spinal cord.

Parasympathetic innervation travels with the *oculomotor nerve* (third cranial nerve), which, on entering the orbit, divides into two branches, the inferior of which contains the parasympathetic fibers bound for the ciliary ganglion and then the eyeball.

Nerve fibers entering the orbit and destined to innervate the eye follow one of two courses. Some proceed directly to the posterior portion of the eye and penetrate the sclera, close to the horizontal meridian; these are the *long posterior ciliary nerves.* Others pass via the ciliary ganglion, which lies near the apex of the orbit between the optic nerve and the lateral rectus muscle. About six to ten *short posterior ciliary nerves* pass from the ciliary ganglion to the eye, where they enter the sclera in a circle around the optic nerve and run forward between the choroid and sclera to form a ciliary plexus in the outer layer of the ciliary body. This plexus is the origin of the nerves of the anterior portion of the eye.

EYELIDS AND CONJUNCTIVA

The anatomy of the eyelids and conjunctiva is important to an understanding of vegetative physiology of the eye because these tissues provide the moisture, lubrication, and protection for the sensitive corneal surface.

The lids join each other at the nasal and temporal corners to form the *inner and outer canthi*. The lids are composed of four major zones. From front to back these are *skin;* a striated muscle called the *orbicularis oculi;* a region of dense fibrous tissue layers called the *tarsi;* and finally the *palpebral conjunctiva,* which forms the lining of the lids.

The tarsi, also called the tarsal plates, are dense fibrous tissues that form the skeleton of the lids. Both upper and lower tarsi are slightly concave so as to fit snugly over the eyeball. The tarsi are attached to the bony orbit by horizontal tendinous *medial and lateral palpebral ligaments.* The deeply recessed location of the insertion of these ligaments ensures that the tarsi will press the lid to the eyeball. In addition to these horizontal ligaments, there is attachment of the orbital borders of the tarsi to the bony orbital margin by the thin membranous *orbital septum.*

Eyelid musculature is compact and complex because it must provide for rapid movement but with little bulk and a relatively large amount of skin stretching. The upper lid has a greater excursion than the lower lid during eye closure in humans. The musculature responsible for eyelid closure is the *orbicularis oculi,* an oval sheet of concentric striated muscle fibers lying between the skin and the fibrous layers of the lid. The lids are opened by action of the *levator palpebrae superioris.* This thin, flat muscle originates at the apex of the orbit and runs forward until it terminates in a thin, broad tendon, the *levator aponeurosis,* which arches over the globe from the nasal to the temporal side. The middle portion of the aponeurosis inserts into the anterior surface of the tarsus and the skin covering the upper lid, while its lateral and medial wings or horns connect to the orbital wall and to the palpebral ligaments. In elevating the eyelid, the levator is aided by the unstriated *Mueller's muscle,* which is a sheet-like branch of the anterior end of the levator muscle running beneath the aponeurosis to an insertion along the upper edge of the tarsus. The lower lid also has a weak counterpart of the muscle of Mueller. (See Figure 1.8.)

Two distinct bundles of orbicularis fibers are not directly involved with lid motion. The lacrimal portions of the orbicularis, or *Horner's muscles,* are placed around the lacrimal canaliculi (see below). These muscles serve to pump tear fluid down the nasolacrimal canal. Another portion of the orbicularis, the *muscle of Riolan,* lies directly under the free borders of the lid and helps to keep them in exact apposition when the eye is closed.

The almond-shaped space between the upper and lower eyelids is the *palpebral fissure.* A thin transparent and continuous mucous membrane, the *conjunctiva,* lines the inside surfaces of the eyelids and covers the anterior surface of the eye, joining the globe at the *limbus.* The conjunctiva connects the edge of the eyelids to the eyeball, and the loose tissue between projects back toward

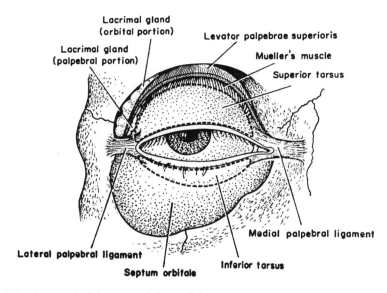

Figure 1.8 Anatomical features of the eyelids.

the equator of the eye; this tissue is folded and doubled back on itself within the *superior and inferior fornices.* The portion lining the lids is the *palpebral con- junctiva* and that over the eye is the *bulbar conjunctiva.* On the nasal side of the eyeball a fold of conjunctiva, the *plica semilunaris,* and the lower lid provide a space capable of holding excess tear fluid. This space is called the *lacrimal lake.*

The moist environment necessary for proper functioning of the cornea is provided by *tear fluid* produced principally by the lacrimal gland. This serous gland lies in the anterior part of the bony orbit and is composed of fine tubules. A number of excretory ducts bring the tears to the conjunctival sac. A small amount of tear fluid is excreted into the conjunctival sac by the accessory lacrimal glands, known as the *glands of Krause, Wolfring,* and *Manz.* An oily substance produced by the *meibomian glands* (of the tarsus) and the *glands of Zeis* in the lids covers the aqueous phase of the tears and serves to reduce the evaporation rate. *Goblet cells* in the conjunctiva supply mucus to keep tears spread over the corneal surface. The tears are usually considered to be about 7 μm in thickness over the corneal surface. Sweat glands (the *glands of Moll*) are also located at the edge of the lids near the roots of the eyelashes.

About 10% of the produced tear fluid is lost by evaporation; the remainder must be continuously drained from the eye. This drainage takes place through two small orifices, the *lacrimal puncta,* at the nasal end of the lid margins. These orifices make contact with the lacrimal lake and draw tears into two narrow channels, the *lacrimal canaliculi.* These canals connect to the *lacrimal sac,* which then leads to the *nasolacrimal duct.* The tears are finally discharged through the nose as part of the nasal secretions.

2

The Aqueous Humor

In a manmade camera, the designer and manufacturer use rigid materials. A rigid glass lens is supported in a metal frame that is in turn attached to a rigid metal box. Photosensitive film is carried inside on a metal sheet at the end of the box opposite the lens. This combination of rigid materials and geometrically exact box-like construction is not available for the eye. The cornea and sclera are thin connective tissues and have little rigidity of their own. The eye therefore achieves its geometrical regularity not by rigidity of its components but by making use of the properties of an inflated spherical membrane.

An almost perfect sphere can be made by blowing a small soap bubble. If a shell is composed of a homogenous, isotropic material, the tension in the wall will be the same at all points in all directions. The surface then assumes a minimum area relative to the enclosed volume, leading to a spherical shape. The eye is not a perfect sphere because the ocular tunic is not a uniform material, but it is sufficiently spherical to satisfy its optical requirements.

If it is accepted from a teleological argument that an inflated spherical shell is the optimum external structure for the eye, the question becomes how to maintain inflation of the sphere. One solution would be to inflate the eye at birth and provide no further inflation process or mechanism; this would be a possible solution (1) if the eye were to remain of constant size during life and (2) if its shell were perfectly impermeable to the internal fluid. Since neither of these conditions is met in the eye, an alternative solution is used. The eye is maintained in its inflated condition by having a liquid, the aqueous humor, continuously produced internally and drained away. The pressure drop across the outflow duct then appears as an internal pressure that is counteracted by the tension in the spherical shell.

Inflow and outflow paths of aqueous humor are traced in this chapter. The tissues and channels involved in aqueous production are described, together with the physical and chemical properties of the fluid produced.

SOURCE OF THE AQUEOUS HUMOR

The primary source of the aqueous humor is the blood flowing in the ciliary arterial system. Bill (1975) estimated that 75 μl/min of plasma flows through the ciliary body of the rabbit, of which 3 μl/min is utilized in the production of aqueous; this decrease of only 4% should have little effect on blood flow. Some of the arteries travel near the surface of the ciliary body and send out fine vessels to form a capillary bed just underneath the two-layer ciliary epithelium, described in Chapter 1. These capillaries have several structural features that appear related to the process of transforming blood plasma into aqueous humor. The capillary walls are tubes of flattened endothelial cells. Where the cell edges overlap, there appears to be a space about 20 nm in width (see *A* in Figure 2.1), but it may be that these spacings are closed at some point because protein molecules smaller than 20 nm are retained within the capillaries. There are also regions in the cell wall where the membrane appears to be perforated or fenestrated (see *B* in Figure 2.1); these fenestrations are not simple pores but are covered with very thin diaphragms that hold back particles 10 nm in diameter or larger. These fenestrations may also be involved in the rapid passage of plasma when aqueous humor must be produced quickly, as when the eye has lost pressure through a penetrating injury (paracentesis).

Three processes have been proposed whereby a clear transparent colorless liquid (the aqueous humor) is produced from the blood. A simple coarse *filtration* will hold back the cellular components and yield the plasma, a slightly yellowish clear liquid of a definite and known composition. Dialysis occurs when a semipermeable membrane is used to separate small (e.g., salt) from large (e.g., protein) particles in solution by diffusion of the former through the membrane. When hydrostatic pressure is used to force both the solvent and small particles across the

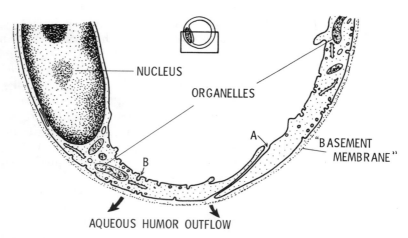

Figure 2.1 Schematic cross-section of a capillary in the ciliary body. (From Davson H [ed.] [1969]: The Eye, Vol. 1. New York, Academic Press.)

semipermeable membrane while the large particles are retained, the process is called *ultrafiltration,* and this has been proposed as a second mechanism in aqueous humor formation. Finally, there is the process of *secretion* in which cells use metabolic energy to do work to pass material, adding and subtracting components and thereby yielding a product possibly quite different from the original.

In early work, Cole (1966) used poisons to inhibit metabolic processes in the ciliary epithelium and suggested that 30% of the aqueous is an ultra-filtrate and 70% is produced by active transport/secretion. Green and Pedersen (1972) and Pedersen and Green (1973) later agreed that ultrafiltration is respon-sible for a substantial portion of aqueous production but reversed the percent-ages, claiming 70% as an ultrafiltrate. Bill (1975), on the other hand, argued that hydrostatic and osmotic pressure conditions across the ciliary epithelium are such that a liquid should flow from the posterior chamber *into* the epithelium; he therefore suggested that active metabolism is primarily responsible for aqueous humor production. Sears (1981) summarized much recent work and concluded that first filtration occurs across the fenestrated capillaries and then aqueous humor is produced by secretion across the two-layered ciliary epithelium.

A simplified schematic of the ciliary epithelium is shown in Figure 2.2. Blood is flowing through the capillaries. The capillary wall holds back blood cells and also perhaps 80% of the plasma proteins—presumably those of high molec-ular weight. The plasma, with about 10% to 20% of its proteins still in solution, fills the extracellular space between these capillaries and the lateral cell walls of the pigmented ciliary epithelium. The plasma layer ends at zonulae occludentes within the apicolateral junction complexes between the two layers of ciliary epithelium. This is believed to be the site of the blood–aqueous barrier. Although some filtration and ultrafiltration may occur between the cells of the ciliary epithelium, it is likely that most if not all of this filtrate is absorbed by the epithelial cells. Compounds are added and subtracted within the ciliary epithelial cells, and a new liquid is secreted at the basoluminal membrane of the nonpig-mented ciliary epithelium, facing the anterior chamber, which is not simply a filtrate of blood plasma.

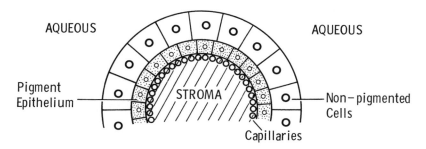

Figure 2.2 Schematic cross-section of the ciliary epithelium showing its relationship to the capillaries and aqueous humor.

Secretion is believed to occur by active transport, which is the movement of material by a process that requires the expenditure of chemical energy derived from a metabolic reaction. The sites of this active transport have been localized at the highly infolded basoluminal membrane of the nonpigmented ciliary epithelial cells (Usukura et al. 1988). Here the production of aqueous humor is a result of the movement of water to restore an osmotic balance upset by the active transport of sodium ion (Na^+) out of the cells. It is likely that Cl^- and/or HCO_3^- move with Na^+ to maintain electroneutrality, and this creates a slightly more concentrated solution on the aqueous side of the cell membranes. These cell membranes are highly permeable to water, facilitating fluid flow, and act like semipermeable barriers so that the osmotic flow of water occurs. This flow is exactly analogous to that taking place in a simple osmometer, as shown in Figure 2.3.

The steady-state height to which a meniscus in such a device will rise is given by van Hoff's osmotic pressure law

$$\Pi = pgh = \Delta c \, RT \tag{2.1}$$

where Π is the osmotic pressure, p is the solution density, h is the height of the meniscus in the tube above the free surface of the external liquid, g is the gravitational constant, R is the universal gas constant 8.32 J/°K-mole (or 8.2×10^{-2} 1-atm/°K-mole), T is the absolute temperature, and Δc is the excess concentration of osmotically active material in the internal solution. *Osmotically active* means that the concentration of material is defined by Equation 2.1 as $\Delta c = \Pi/RT =$

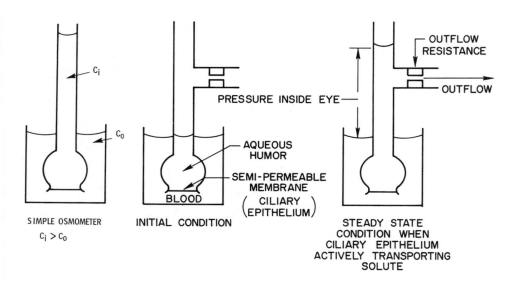

Figure 2.3 An osmometer arranged to illustrate osmotic flow across the ciliary epithelium.

pgh/*RT.* If Δ*c* equals 1 Osm/liter, the osmotic pressure is 22.4 atmospheres. A solution that has an excess concentration of 1 mOsm/liter will have an osmotic pressure of almost 17 mmHg.

The cells of the ciliary epithelium use metabolic energy to transfer osmotically active material into the aqueous humor, equivalent to moving this material from the outside to the inside of the osmometer shown in Figure 2.3. The osmotic pressure difference then causes a passive movement of water from the outside to the inside as well. In the simple osmometer shown in Figure 2.3, the internal solution rises in the vertical tube until the hydrostatic pressure head counterbalances the force driving water inward across the semipermeable membrane, then the flow of water stops. In the case of the ciliary epithelium, a chemical process continues to move osmotically active solute into the osmometer, necessitating a drain in our model if pressure is to be held constant. A side arm can therefore be installed and the solution inside the osmometer can be continually drawn away once a certain pressure is achieved. As long as the ciliary body can do metabolic work and fresh blood is supplied to one side, fluid will be produced and then drained away.

The osmotic pressure produced by active transport of Na^+ that causes aqueous production is partially offset by the colloid osmotic pressure, known also as the oncotic pressure, of the large plasma proteins, which cannot get into the aqueous humor. The effect of oncotic pressure can be demonstrated by the rapid reduction of intraocular pressure that occurs with intravenous injection of mannitol. Mannitol increases the oncotic pressure, drawing water out of the anterior chamber and vitreous body and into the capillaries.

CHEMISTRY

Chemical analysis of aqueous humor shows clearly that it is not simply blood plasma. It is a clear solution of about the same density and viscosity as water; specific gravity varies from 1.0034 to 1.0036 (Hogan et al. 1971). Aqueous humor, for instance, has a very much lower protein content than plasma, as shown in Table 2.1. Because protein molecules are large enough to scatter light (the Tyndall effect) and are therefore colloids by definition, the protein content is also the *colloid content*. Noncolloids are the dissolved solids that give an absolutely clear solution—one in which a beam of light would not be seen. The noncolloid content of rabbit aqueous humor, compared to plasma, is given in

Table 2.1 Comparison of Protein Content of Plasma and Aqueous Humor for Human and Rabbit*

Species	Plasma	Aqueous Humor
Human	6000–7000 mg/100 ml	5–16 mg/100 ml
Rabbit	6000–7000 mg/100 ml	50 mg/100 ml

*After Davson H (ed.)(1969): The Eye, Vol. 1. New York, Academic Press.

Table 2.2. Although cursory inspection suggests similarity, careful review indicates clear differences that are inconsistent with aqueous being simply a filtrate. For example, the concentrations of ascorbate and pyruvate are much higher in the rabbit aqueous humor than in the plasma, and those of urea and glucose are much lower.

The presence of large organic molecules in aqueous cannot be explained by filtration or ultrafiltration or by the active transport of Na^+. The entry of these substances has been the subject of much debate. Ascorbate particularly illustrates active transport, as its concentration in the aqueous humor increases directly with changes in the plasma until a saturation level of about 5 mg/100 ml (at a plasma level of about 50 mg/100 ml) is reached (Kinsey 1947). The metabolic consumption of glucose and production of lactate by the surrounding ocular tissues at least partially account for the differences between aqueous and plasma concentrations of these substances. Ross (1951, 1952) claimed to have demonstrated the active transport of glucose, but his work could not be duplicated. The fact that xylose, galactose, and 3-methyl glucose penetrate equally well would indicate that there is not an active transport mechanism peculiar to glucose. A diffusion process in which glucose is carried across the cells, called *facilitated diffusion,* has been invoked to explain the transport of glucose. Freddo and co-workers (1990) additionally presented evidence for a direct diffusion of macromolecules, on the order of albumin in size, from the ciliary and iridal processes into the aqueous. Finally, the active transport of Na^+ favors the migration of anions in the same direction, so lactate may preferentially move toward the aqueous.

Table 2.2   Comparison of Noncolloid Content of Rabbit Plasma and Aqueous Humor*

Component	Concentration (mM/kg water†)	
	Plasma	Aqueous Humor
Na	151.50	143.50
K	4.72	4.55
Ca	2.60	1.70
Mg	1.00	0.78
Cl	108.00	109.50
HCO_3	27.40	33.60
Lactate	4.30	7.40
Pyruvate	0.22	0.66
Ascorbate	0.02	0.96
Urea	9.10	7.00
Glucose	8.30	6.90

*From Davson H (ed.) (1969): The Eye, Vol 1. New York, Academic Press.
†mM, millimole, 1/1000 gm mole

Further evidence that aqueous is not just a filtrate or ultrafiltrate of blood plasma—plasma minus most of its colloids—might be offered by a comparison of a dialysate of blood plasma to the known composition of aqueous humor, but species differences and technical difficulties in analysis have not permitted a definitive conclusion on this basis. Davson (1956), however, carried out a very careful analysis in which he compared the *distribution ratios* of several components of aqueous humor to those of a dialysate of plasma. The distribution ratio (R_{aq}) of a component of aqueous humor is defined as

$$R_{aq} = \frac{c_{aq}}{c_{plasma}} \tag{2.2}$$

where c_{aq} is the concentration of the component in the aqueous and c_{plasma} is its concentration in the plasma. Similarly, the distribution ratio of a component of the dialysate is

$$R_{dial} = \frac{c_{dial}}{c_{plasma}} \tag{2.3}$$

The results of Davson's work are shown in Table 2.3. Although the differences in R values are very small for most components, the accuracy with which these values were measured was sufficient to indicate that these differences were significant and again demonstrates that aqueous humor is not simply a dialysate of plasma.

Why does aqueous humor fail to show a higher Na^+ content than the plasma in Table 2.2 if there is active Na^+ transport into the anterior chamber? The

Table 2.3 Comparison of R_{aq} and R_{dial} (Defined by Equations 2.2 and 2.3)*

Component	R_{ag}	R_{dial}
Na	0.96	0.945
K	0.955	0.96
Mg	0.78	0.80
Ca	0.58	0.65
Cl	1.015	1.04
HCO$_3$	1.26	1.04
H$_2$CO$_3$	1.29	1.00
Phosphate	0.58	—
Glucose	0.86	0.97
Urea	0.97	—
Ascorbate	18.50	—
Lactate	1.70	—

*After Davson H (1956). Physiology of the Ocular and Cerebrospinal Fluids. Boston, Little, Brown.

osmotic effect induced by active transport is restricted to a thin film of freshly secreted, concentrated fluid immediately adjacent to the nonpigmented ciliary epithelium luminal membrane. Sodium ion (Na^+) is continuously diffusing away from this zone and being absorbed into the vitreous body. It may not be possible to see the conditions existent for osmotic flow across the ciliary epithelium from a gross chemical analysis of aqueous humor such as presented in Table 2.2.

In addition to the solids listed in Tables 2.1 and 2.2, two important gases are in solution in the aqueous humor: oxygen and carbon dioxide. Oxygen is supplied by the blood flowing through the arterial system of the ciliary body and iris. Carbon dioxide is a product of cellular metabolism in the cells of the ciliary body, iris, lens epithelium, and corneal endothelium. Blood flowing in the venous system of the ciliary body and iris carries away the carbon dioxide.

Before presenting the data on oxygen content of the aqueous humor, it is necessary to discuss the units that are used. One of the most common and convenient ways of expressing the oxygen concentration in a liquid is to state the oxygen content of a gas mixture that would be in equilibrium with the oxygen dissolved in the liquid. This is called the *partial pressure* or *oxygen tension* of the liquid. (The term *tension* is more common than the term *partial pressure* in the biological literature and will be used throughout this book.) For example, the aqueous humor of an air-breathing rabbit has been found to be in equilibrium with a gas that has an oxygen content about one-third that of air. The pressure of the standard atmosphere is 760 mmHg, that is, it will support a column of mercury 760 mm high. By Dalton's law of partial pressure, the pressure of oxygen in air is quite close to the volume fraction of oxygen in air, about 0.20, multiplied by the total pressure. Therefore, the oxygen tension of air is 0.20×760 mmHg, or 152 mmHg. The oxygen tension of air-breathing rabbit aqueous is then approximately 0.33×152 mmHg = 50 mmHg.

The amount of dissolved oxygen can be known only if both the tension and the solubility of oxygen in aqueous humor are known. The relationship between tension, oxygen content, and solubility is known as *Henry's law* and can be stated as

$$c = kP \qquad (2.4)$$

where c is the dissolved oxygen concentration, k is its solubility, and P is the oxygen tension in solution. If aqueous humor is assumed to have the same k as pure water, then the aqueous humor of the air-breathing rabbit at 39°C has 0.0018 ml of gaseous oxygen (when measured at 1 atmosphere and 0°C—this condition will be used in all subsequent statements of dissolved gas content) dissolved in each milliliter.

Arterial blood is the source of oxygen in the aqueous humor. Experiments on rabbits show that aqueous humor oxygen tension is in the range of 25 to 75 mmHg while air is breathed but increases directly with the oxygen content of the breathed gas reaching 100 to 300 mmHg for an animal breathing pure oxygen (Heald and Langham 1956; Jacobi 1968; Kleinstein et al. 1981).

The carbon dioxide tension in the aqueous humor is about the same as that of oxygen (by coincidence), namely 50 mmHg. The solubility of carbon dioxide in water, however, is much greater than that of oxygen. Aqueous humor therefore has about 0.043 ml of carbon dioxide per milliliter.

The hydrogen ion content, known as pH, of the aqueous humor is 7.60, compared to 7.40 for the blood plasma (note, pH is $-\log H^+$ concentration by convention).

RATE OF PRODUCTION OF AQUEOUS HUMOR

The rate of aqueous production must be equal to the rate of its drainage or the eye would either swell or shrink with time. However, just because these rates are equal does not mean they are unimportant to the condition of the eye. Intraocular pressure, counterbalanced by the tension in the outer tunic, is determined quantitatively by the product of the flow rate and the resistance to outflow. Production rates have been studied by a variety of methods for this reason. The chemical tracer methods of flow rate measurement are described here; procedures that require measurement of intraocular pressure are discussed in Chapter 3. Bill (1975) has presented an excellent review of the entire field of fluid dynamics and blood circulation in the eye.

The rate of aqueous humor production cannot be measured by simply tapping the eye with a calibrated tube as shown in Figure 2.4. If the leveling bulb is raised to give a pressure in the calibrated tube above the intraocular pressure, fluid will be driven from the tube into the eye until the internal pressure matches that

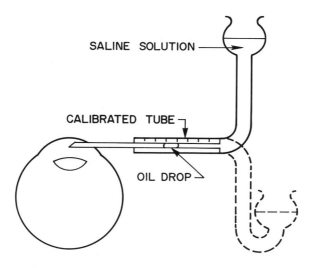

Figure 2.4 Demonstration of an attempt to make a direct measurement of aqueous flow rate.

caused by the raised leveling bulb, and then inflow will stop. If the pressure produced by the leveling bulb is below that in the eye, the eye will shrink and the flow observed in the calibrated tube will come from the collapse of the eye and any ongoing aqueous production, until again the pressure in the eye equals that produced by the leveling bulb. If the pressure imposed by the leveling bulb matches that in the eye, a bubble of oil within the calibrated tube will not move and therefore no flow rate will be observed. Under all conditions of the leveling bulb, the normal outflow paths for aqueous humor in the eye are functioning and so movement of fluid in the calibrated tube is controlled by pressure differences between the leveling bulb and the eye and has no relation to aqueous humor flow rate.

Instead of tapping the eye, a chemical tracer that will quickly mix with the entire volume of aqueous humor to give a solution of known concentration can be injected into the anterior chamber. The tracer will drain out with the normal outflow of aqueous humor. The rate of disappearance of the injected chemical from the anterior chamber is then a measure of the outflow rate of aqueous humor. The major requirements of this method are that the injection process does not disturb the eye's normal production and drainage mechanisms and that the tracer does not leave the anterior chamber except with the aqueous humor. For example, if the tracer absorbs onto the iris or cornea, then the amount leaving with the aqueous is not known. The use of tracers is so universal in the study of physiological fluid production and drainage that a detailed description of this technique is warranted.

Let S be the mass of tracer, either a dye or radioactive material, dissolved in aqueous humor. The rate at which the amount of tracer in the anterior chamber is changing is $-dS/dt$. The negative sign here shows that tracer is leaving the anterior chamber. The tracer is carried away by a flow rate of F ml/min of a solution of concentration c_{aq} gm/ml. Therefore, the rate at which tracer is removed is also Fc_{aq}. These two statements can be mathematically equated:

$$\frac{-dS}{dt} = Fc_{aq} \qquad (2.5)$$

The definition of concentration in the aqueous humor, c_{aq}, is

$$c_{aq} = \frac{S}{V_a} \qquad (2.6)$$

where V_a is the chamber volume. By rearrangement of Equation 2.6 we have

$$S = V_a c_{aq} \qquad (2.7)$$

Equation 2.5 can now be written

$$-\frac{dS}{dt} = -\frac{d(V_a c_{aq})}{dt} = -\frac{V_a dc_{aq}}{dt} = -Fc_{aq} \qquad (2.8)$$

because we assume that V_a remains constant during the measurement. If we identify the concentration of tracer in the aqueous humor immediately on injection as c_{aq}°, we have the integration limits on Equation 2.8. The integral form of Equation 2.8 is

$$\int_{c_{aq}^{\circ}}^{c_{aq}} \frac{dc_{aq}}{c_{aq}} = -\left(\frac{F}{V_a}\right)\int_0^t dt \qquad (2.9)$$

Since $dc/c = \log_e c$, Equation 2.9 integrates to

$$\int_{c_{aq}^{\circ}}^{c_{aq}} \frac{dc_{aq}}{c_{aq}} = \log_e c_{aq} - \log_e c_{aq}^{\circ} = \log_e \frac{c_{aq}}{c_{aq}^{\circ}} = -\frac{Ft}{V_a} \qquad (2.10)$$

or

$$c_{aq} = c_{aq}^{\circ}\, exp\left\{\frac{-Ft}{V_a}\right\} \qquad (2.11)$$

Equation 2.11 shows that there will be an exponential decrease of tracer concentration with time.

Noting that the relation between $\log_e$ and $\log_{10}$ is $\log_e x = 2.303 \log_{10} x$, we can write

$$\log \frac{c_{aq}}{c_{aq}^{\circ}} = -\frac{Ft}{2.303}\, V_a \qquad (2.12)$$

where the symbol "log" refers to log to the base 10.

Equation 2.12 indicates that a plot of c_{aq}/c_{aq}° on the log scale and t on the arithmetic scale of semilogarithmic paper will produce a straight line. The slope of this line will be given by

$$\Delta\frac{\left(\log\frac{c_{aq}}{c_{aq}^{\circ}}\right)}{\Delta t} = -\frac{F}{2.303}\, V_a \qquad (2.13)$$

If the time for a tenfold drop in c_{aq} is called t_1, then we have

$$\Delta\frac{\left(\log\frac{c_{aq}}{c_{aq}^{\circ}}\right)}{t_1} = \frac{\left(\log\frac{1}{10}\right)}{t_1} = -\frac{1}{t_1} \qquad (2.14)$$

and therefore

$$\frac{F}{V_a} = \frac{2.303}{t_1} \qquad (2.15)$$

The term F/V_a has units of 1/time and is simply the fraction of fluid that leaves each minute. This fractional flow rate will hereafter be called f_a.

The tracer method described above has some serious disadvantages when applied to the anterior chamber. First, the process of inserting a needle and injecting tracer raises the intraocular pressure. Pulling the needle abruptly out of the eye also lowers intraocular pressure. Such pressure changes are known to interfere with aqueous humor production and may invalidate the data collected. Davson and Spaziani (1960) also noted that there is little likelihood of immediate and complete mixing of tracer and aqueous humor on injection, although this is assumed in the mathematics above. Their study of the tracer method suggested that mixing was indeed inadequate and that calculated flow rates were too high by about a factor of 10.

Maurice (1959) tried an alternative approach to the tracer method. He injected very small quantities of radioactive protein into the vitreous humor of a living rabbit. He immediately held the whole eye of the animal near a radioactivity counter and obtained a number for all of the tracer in the globe. The eye was enucleated after a known time interval, the aqueous and vitreous humors were separated, and the radioactivity of each was measured. Mathematical analysis of this data is made as follows. The fraction of anterior chamber fluid flowing out of the eye each minute is f_a as above. The volume leaving the eye in a minute is $f_a V_a$, where V_a is the volume of the anterior chamber as defined above. The amount of tracer leaving the eye in a minute is $f_a V_a c_a$, where c_a is the concentration of radioactive tracer in the aqueous humor. The radioactive tracer in the aqueous humor came by diffusion from the vitreous humor. If it is assumed that the tracer does not leave the vitreous by any other pathway, then in the *steady state* the rate of loss of tracer from the vitreous is equal to the rate that the tracer is carried away by outflow of aqueous humor. Stated mathematically, that is

$$f_a V_a c_a = f_v V_v c_v \tag{2.16a}$$

or

$$f_a = f_v \left(\frac{V_v}{V_a}\right) / \left(\frac{c_a}{c_v}\right) \tag{2.16b}$$

where c_v is the concentration of tracer in the vitreous humor of volume V_v and f_v is the *fraction* of the tracer in the vitreous that leaves each minute.

Equation 2.16 is true at all times during the steady state. The term f_v was calculated from the rate of loss of radioactivity for the whole eye. This calculation ignores the volume of the anterior chamber relative to that of the vitreous, but the error is only about 9% since the ratio of volumes V_a/V_v is only 0.35 ml/4 ml in the rabbit. The ratio c_a/c_v was obtained from the ratio of radioactivity in the aqueous and vitreous humors when the eye was later opened. The remaining term f_a in Equation 2.16 could then be calculated and was found to be 0.0085 min^{-1}. This means that 0.85% of the volume of the anterior chamber is leaving per minute. Since the known volume of the chamber is 0.35 ml, the outflow rate must be $F_a = f_a V_a$, or 0.0085/min × 0.35 ml = 0.003 ml/min. Since aqueous humor must not increase or decrease in volume in the steady state, the rate of production must also be 0.003 ml/min.

To avoid the need to inject tracer directly into the eye, Barany and Kinsey (1949) introduced the tracer into the bloodstream and observed its disappearance from the eye. The tracer p-aminohippurate, when injected into the blood, gives only a temporary high concentration of this material in the plasma because it is rapidly removed by the kidneys. During the time the concentration of p-amino-hippurate is high in the plasma, a large amount will appear in the aqueous humor. Aqueous humor, however, as we have seen above, is not a direct part of the circulating blood plasma and therefore the concentration of p-aminohippurate will remain relatively high in the aqueous after its concentration in the plasma has been returned to a negligible level by the action of the kidneys. Under these conditions, there is a tracer-labeled solution in the anterior chamber that is slowly being replaced by tracer-free freshly produced aqueous humor. The tracer can only leave with the outward flow of aqueous humor.

The experimental procedure was as follows. One hour after injection of p-aminohippurate into the bloodstream of a rabbit, the animal was anesthetized, and one eye was removed. The aqueous humor was withdrawn from this eye, and the p-aminohippurate concentration was determined. An additional hour later, the second eye was removed from the still-living animal, and the tracer concentration in the aqueous of this eye was also measured. The difference in concentrations between the two eyes allowed the flow of aqueous humor to be calculated, assuming that both eyes had the same concentration when the first eye was removed. Barany and Kinsey (1949) found that aqueous was being replaced at 1.2% to 1.4%/min. This gives a rabbit aqueous humor production rate of 0.0042 to 0.0045 ml/min for an anterior chamber volume of 0.35 ml.

Fluorescein dye can be used as the tracer in human studies because its concentration in the aqueous humor can be determined *in vivo* by noninvasive optical means. Goldmann (1950) injected this dye and found that the flow rate of aqueous into the human eye was 1.1% ± 0.22% of the anterior chamber volume per minute. This means that about half the aqueous is exchanged per hour.

Instead of introducing fluorescein into the blood as did Goldmann (1950), Jones and Maurice (1966) used the direct migration of fluorescein inward across the cornea in an electric field (iontophoresis) to introduce this tracer into the aqueous humor. They found a similar figure for the flow rate of human aqueous: 1.53% ± 0.11% of the anterior chamber volume per minute.

OUTFLOW PATH OF AQUEOUS HUMOR

There is a clearly defined circular channel in the limbus of primate eyes, the *canal of Schlemm,* that forms the major outflow path for aqueous humor. This canal is lined with a layer of endothelial cells. A *trabecular meshwork* of connective tissue covered by endothelial cells separates the canal of Schlemm and the anterior chamber. Aqueous humor that passes from the anterior chamber to the lumen of Schlemm's canal must percolate through the trabecular meshwork and through the endothelial lining of the canal. The resistance to flow presented by these tissues together with the aqueous humor production rate determine the pressure that will be present in the eye. The exact structure of this combined bed of fibers and cells is not known, but it is known that particles at least as large as 1.5 to 3.0 μm can pass through. Some investigators believe that this is evidence for a pore structure, but this view is disputed because large particles such as red blood

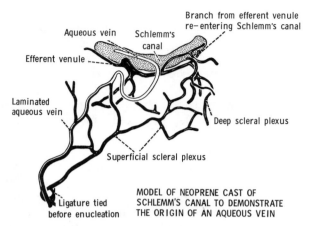

Branch from efferent venule
re-entering Schlemm's canal

Aqueous vein   Schlemm's
canal

Efferent venule

Laminated
aqueous vein

Deep scleral plexus

Superficial scleral plexus

Ligature tied
before enucleation

MODEL OF NEOPRENE CAST OF
SCHLEMM'S CANAL TO DEMONSTRATE
THE ORIGIN OF AN AQUEOUS VEIN

Figure 2.5 Drawing made from a neoprene rubber cast of Schlemm's canal and the aqueous veins. (After Ashton N [1951]: Anatomical study of Schlemm's canal and aqueous veins by means of neoprene casts. Br. J. Opthalmol. 35:291–303.)

cells (about 8 μm in diameter) pass through other tissues of the body without the presence of demonstrable pores.

The fluid collected by the canal of Schlemm is delivered to the episcleral venous system by a special set of vessels called the *aqueous veins,* which originate directly on the canal. These then join the superficial scleral venous plexus, but without penetration for a short distance (a laminated vein). The lumens finally do join and two veins become one (Figure 2.5).

Schlemm's canal is undoubtedly the major outflow route for aqueous humor. About 20% of the total outflow of fluid, however, may occur by simple percolation through the outer tunic of the eye into the orbit, where it is absorbed into the lymphatic system. Bill (1964) has called this the *unconventional outflow path* or the *uveoscleral route.* Fatt and Hedbys (1970b) showed that there would be sufficient outflow of fluid through the loose choroid meshwork at normal intraocular pressure to account for 20% of aqueous humor drainage. Kleinstein and Fatt (1977) directly measured the outflow of aqueous humor across rabbit sclera and confirmed that 10% to 20% of aqueous could drain by this trans-scleral route. There is also evidence that aqueous humor moves through or around the vitreous body and then outward through the retina, pigment epithelium, choroid, and sclera (Fatt and Shantinath 1971). Trans-scleral flow of aqueous humor is therefore a substantial if not major part of the outflow system of the eye.

3

The Intraocular Pressure

The internal, or intraocular, pressure (abbreviated IOP or P_{ioc}) of the eye is of interest to both the physiologist and the clinician. To the physiologist IOP is a manifestation of those biophysical and biochemical processes that produce and drain the intraocular fluids. These processes include passive osmotic pressure and active transport. Both are lively areas of study in physiology. To the ophthalmic clinician IOP is of deep concern because abnormally high IOP, a serious medical condition called *glaucoma,* can lead to irreversible blindness. Two forms of glaucoma are recognized. In *angle-closure* glaucoma the iris is pushed against the posterior surface of the corneal–scleral junction (see Figure 1.2), thereby blocking access of aqueous humor to Schlemm's canal. Since Schlemm's canal is the major outflow route for aqueous humor from the eye, angle-closure glaucoma leads to a rapid and painful increase in IOP. A painless but common form of glaucoma known as *open-angle* glaucoma can also lead to blindness. In open-angle glaucoma there is a slow rise in IOP. The increase in IOP is a result of either a slowly increasing aqueous humor production rate or a slowly developing increase in liquid flow resistance in the aqueous humor outflow pathway.

METHODS OF MEASUREMENT

Before discussing IOP and the physiological factors that control it, the methods of measurement must be introduced. By far the simplest method would be to perform a direct tap of the eye, but this is suitable only for nonhuman research purposes. A direct tap to the fluid in the eye is equivalent to applying an air-pressure gauge to an automobile or bicycle tire, but there are some significant differences. First, the eye is filled with an incompressible fluid, essentially water, that should not be removed in the process of making the measurement. The loss of even a small amount of fluid, removed to operate a pressure-measuring device, could cause a large drop in IOP. Second, this intraocular fluid is continuously produced and drained away.

Modern electronic pressure transducers, however, require very little fluid to activate their mechanisms, perhaps only 5 µl to record a pressure of 100 mmHg.

The rabbit eye typically has an IOP of about 20 mmHg and an aqueous production rate of about 2.5 μl/min, and IOP can be measured in only 30 seconds. A transducer connected to a fine hypodermic needle inserted through the cornea into the anterior chamber could therefore tap the fluid in the eye and record IOP with minimal trauma or loss of fluid that might otherwise disturb such a measurement.

Although a direct pressure tap can now be almost atraumatic, this method would not be clinically suitable for routine use on human patients. Because some pain is involved in this procedure, anesthesia is required, and there are risks of damage to the internal structures, scarring, and infection in any penetration of the eye. Clinical measurements of IOP are therefore made by indirect methods, through the use of an instrument called a *tonometer*.

Henson (1983) has given a useful description of clinical tonometers, which generally fall into two classes. *Indentation* or *impression* tonometers, of which the Schiøtz (invented in 1905) is the most common example, measure the depth of indentation made by a plunger of known weight placed onto the cornea. *Applanation* tonometers (e.g., the Goldmann tonometer), on the other hand, measure the force required to flatten a known area of the corneal surface.

SCHIØTZ TONOMETRY

The Schiøtz tonometer, shown in Figure 3.1, is a simple, inexpensive, and reliable instrument. It has several disadvantages, however. First, a topical anesthetic must be applied to the eye prior to measurement because otherwise such indentation would be too painful for patients to tolerate. This is a relatively minor problem; other forms of tonometry also require a topical anesthetic. A more important problem is the absence of a simple equation, derivable from physical principles, that relates the measured depth of indentation to IOP. An empirically determined calibration curve—with certain assumptions—must be used instead. And finally, the IOP read by the Schiøtz tonometer depends on the physical properties of the cornea. As these properties can change with age or disease, the calibration of the Schiøtz tonometer can change. Despite these disadvantages, it has been a widely used clinical device for measuring IOP.

The Schiøtz instrument is essentially two levers used to magnify the movement of the plunger (P in Figure 3.1) as it indents the cornea. One division of movement of the pointer (X) on the Schiøtz scale represents a plunger movement of 0.05 mm relative to the footplate (F). A recently developed modification of this instrument replaces the pointer with a digital readout, and the measurement value is held after the device is removed from the eye. Although one would expect that zero indentation would correspond to a zero scale reading, actually the test block sets scale zero at a plunger protrusion of 0.05 mm beyond the footplate. The establishment of a zero scale reading at 0.05-mm indentation is based on Schiøtz's belief that there is a viscous indentation of the plunger into soft epithelium of this magnitude unrelated to IOP. The test block allows this protrusion of the plunger by having a slightly greater radius of curvature than the footplate (16 vs. 15 mm,

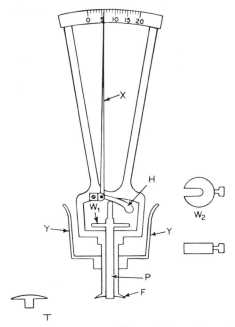

Figure 3.1 Schiøtz tonometer. Parts are as follows: *F*, footplate; *H*, lever arm resting on plunger; *P*, plunger; *T*, test block to zero indicator arm; W_1, weight in place on plunger; W_2, spare weight; *X*, indicator arm; *Y*, frame to be held between fingers by the operator. (From Davson H [ed.] [1969] The Eye, Vol. 1. New York, Academic Press.)

respectively) for the same chord diameter, thereby setting this protrusion as a zero scale reading.

The operating principle of the Schiøtz tonometer is shown in Figure 3.2. A vertical plunger of weight *W* deforms the cornea because its applied force *mg* (*m* is mass and *g* is the gravitational constant; the Schiøtz tonometer would require the use of larger weights if used on the moon) is greater than the counteractive force *A* (IOP), where *A* is the area over which the indentation is effective. The Schiøtz tonometer weighs about 11 gm, increasing to a total weight of 16.5 gm with the normally used 5.5-gm addition (7.5- and 10.0-gm additions are also available). The intraocular fluid displaced by this indentation is incompressible and so must make room for itself in the eye by extending the elastic tunic, that is, by stretching the sclera. Some of the displaced fluid can also leave the globe by the usual outflow routes discussed in Chapter 2. Very little fluid, however, can leave the eye during the very short time that the tonometer is resting on the cornea in clinical application. Almost immediately after applying the tonometer to the eye, the pressure generated in the eye by the stretched sclera exactly balances the force exerted by the plunger, and no further indentation takes place. Extra weights are provided with the Schiøtz tonometer, and these can be added to the plunger to give the additional indentation force required to measure high IOPs (see below).

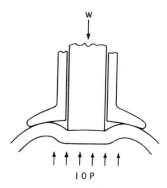

Figure 3.2 Schematic showing indentation of the cornea when plunger of weight W is placed on eye of intraocular pressure IOP. (From Davson H [ed.] [1969]: The Eye, Vol. 1. New York, Academic Press.)

If the Schiøtz tonometer is allowed to remain on the eye for several minutes, the fluid displaced by indentation will eventually escape by the usual outflow paths and the pressure will fall to what it was before the indentation began. The scale reading will increase as the plunger sinks deeper with decreasing IOP during this time period. Since maintaining the tonometer on the eye is uncomfortable for the patient and time-consuming for the operator, and as the time for the return to original pressure is highly variable, it is usual practice to take only the initial indentation measurement and then include in the tonometer's calibration a correction for the increase in observed IOP due to application of the instrument to the eye.

The construction of the Schiøtz calibration chart involves use of the *ocular rigidity* concept and is therefore worth discussing in detail. The theory of ocular rigidity was introduced by Friedenwald (1937), who assumed that the fractional increase in volume, $\Delta V/V$, of an eye would be proportional to the accompanying fractional increase in pressure, $\Delta P/P$. This statement can be written in the form of a differential equation as

$$\frac{dP}{P} = k\frac{dV}{V} \tag{3.1}$$

where k is a proportionality constant. The change in ocular volume is very small in tonometry. Friedenwald chose to assume that the original volume V remained constant and therefore wrote his equation as

$$\frac{dP}{P} = K'\,dV \tag{3.2}$$

where $K' = k/V$. Even if the proportionality constant k, which may be a function of tissue properties, is truely constant, it is clear that the K' term will be a function of ocular volume.

When Equation 3.2 is integrated, the result is

$$\log_e P_2 - \log_e P_1 = K' \, (V_2 - V_1) \qquad (3.3)$$

$\log_e$ is the natural logarithm where e is denoted as 2.718; then $\log_e 2.718 = 1$, whereas in common logarithms $\log 10 = 1$.

Noting that $\log_e P_2 - \log_e P_1 = \log_e P_2/P_1$, and allowing $V_2 - V_1 = \Delta V$, Equation 3.3 may be rewritten as

$$\log_e \frac{P_2}{P_1} = K' \, \Delta V \qquad (3.4)$$

Since logarithms based on 10 ("common" logarithms) are more familiar than those based on e, it is convenient to change Equation 3.4 to the base 10 by noting that $\log x = (1/2.303) \log_e x$, where the logarithm to base 10 will have no subscript. Equation 3.4 then becomes

$$\log \frac{P_2}{P_1} = \left(\frac{K'}{2.303}\right) \Delta V \qquad (3.5)$$

If we let $K'/2.303$ be K, then we have developed the well-known Friedenwald equation

$$\log \frac{P_2}{P_1} = K \, \Delta V \qquad (3.6)$$

where P_1 is the initial IOP, P_2 is the new pressure, and ΔV is the change in ocular volume associated with P_2.

The term K in Equation 3.6 is called the *ocular rigidity* by convention. Note that K is not the true proportionality constant (k) between fractional changes in volume and pressure but is closely related to this constant by the equation $K = (k/2.303 \, V)$. Ocular rigidity is sometimes called *scleral rigidity* because the sclera is a large fraction ($13/14$) of the globe in humans; when an internal pressure increase stretches the eye, it is largely the sclera that is stretched.

Equation 3.6 forms the basis for relating the depth of penetration of the Schiøtz tonometer plunger, observed as a reading on its scale, to the pressure in the eye *before* the tonometer was placed on the cornea. Let P_2 be the pressure in the eye with the tonometer in place indenting the cornea, and let ΔV be the volume of this indentation. The quantity desired is P_1 and is given by rearrangement of Equation 3.6 to

$$\log P_1 = \log P_2 - K\Delta V \qquad (3.7)$$

If P_2 is the measured quantity, and ΔV and K are known, then equation 3.7 will allow determination of P_1, assumed to be the true IOP.

It is first necessary to relate the Schiøtz tonometer scale readings to the IOP. Since the Schiøtz tonometer is simply a device for measuring depth of indentation of the cornea by a plunger under a fixed force, this device can be calibrated by fixing the pressure in an eye, placing a Schiøtz tonometer on the cornea, and then observing the resultant measurement. If a freshly enucleated human eye is connected directly to a leveling bulb reservoir, as shown in Figure 3.3, and there is no other way for fluid to enter or exit, only the height of the leveling bulb sets the pressure within the eye. The presence or absence of the tonometer on the eye will not affect the pressure under this condition. A series of Schiøtz readings (called R) may then be made for a group of corresponding IOPs (values of P_2 as the tonometer is on the eye), set by the height of the leveling bulb. Friedenwald found that the relation between tonometer weight W, pressure P_2, and scale reading R was

$$\frac{W}{P_2} = a + bR \tag{3.8}$$

where a and b are constants that can be obtained from a plot of the data. The numerical values of the constants a and b used in Schiøtz tonometry are given in Table 3.1. These constants were used in constructing Friedenwald's 1955 Calibration for the Schiøtz Tonometer, shown here as Table 3.2 on page 41.

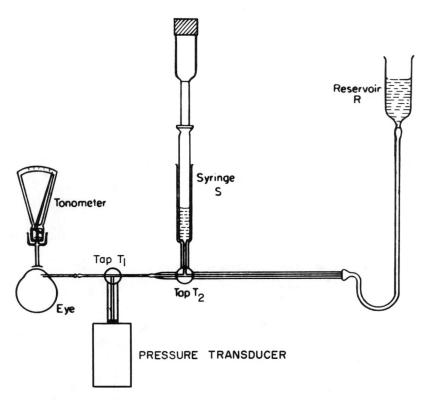

Figure 3.3 Schematic of apparatus used to relate Schiøtz tonometer readings to intraocular pressure. (From Gloster J [1965]: Tonometry and Tonography, Vol. 5, No. 4. International Ophthalmology Clinics. Boston, Little, Brown.)

Table 3.1   Summary of Schiøtz Tonometry Constants

Weight	A	B
5.5 gm	0.107	0.0138
7.5 gm	0.107	0.0138
10.0 gm	0.107	0.0138

Use of the experimentally determined values of a and b in Equation 3.8 allows determination of the equilibrium or long-term pressure, P_2, in an eye while the Schiøtz tonometer is resting on the eye. In clinical practice, we are most interested, however, in P_1 (the pressure in the eye *without* the *increase* in pressure due to the presence of the tonometer on the eye). If K is known, if the relationship between a change in volume and the related increase in pressure can be determined, and if the indentation volume caused by the tonometer could be measured, Equation 3.7 may then be used to correct the observed pressure (P_2) to that which would be present in the absence of the indentation (P_1).

Gloster (1965) used the apparatus shown in Figure 3.4 to determine the relationship between the Schiøtz scale reading and the volume of indentation. The leveling-bulb reservoir established a pressure under the excised cornea that was not changed by the tonometer. On application of the tonometer to the test cornea, a volume of fluid was displaced that moved a bubble trapped in the graduated tube. Figure 3.5 shows Gloster's results: the change in volume or fluid displaced for several scale readings of the tonometer with the 7.5-gm weight attached to the plunger for six sample human corneas.

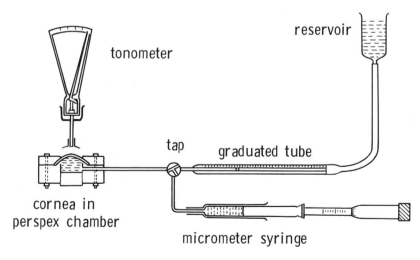

Figure 3.4   Schematic of apparatus used to relate the Schiøtz scale reading to the volume of corneal indentation. (From Gloster J [1965]: Tonometry and Tonography, Vol. 5, No. 4. International Ophthalmology Clinics. Boston, Little, Brown.)

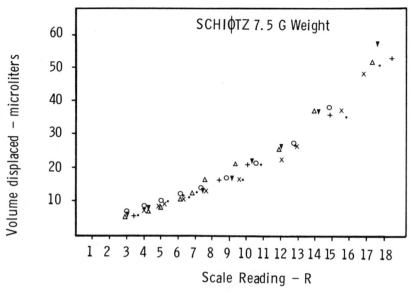

Figure 3.5 Relationship between volume of indentation of the Schiøtz plunger and reading on the Schiøtz scale. (From Gloster J [1965]: Tonometry and Tonography, Vol. 5, No. 4. International Ophthalmology Clinics. Boston, Little, Brown.)

After obtaining a scale reading (R in Figure 3.5) on the Schiøtz tonometer, Equation 3.8 can be used to calculate P_2, and then Figure 3.5 gives ΔV. If ocular rigidity K is known, Equation 3.7 can be used to calculate the pressure (P_1) in the eye before it is raised by the application of the Schiøtz tonometer to the cornea.

To determine K experimentally, the stopcocks shown in Figure 3.3 are arranged so that IOP (the eye, human or animal, may be that of a living animal or perhaps one that has been freshly enucleated) can be observed. The initial pressure is first set by the leveling bulb. The stopcock is then turned to exclude the leveling bulb but to include both the syringe and the electronic pressure transducer so that changes in pressure can be immediately measured when small, known volumes (5 to 10 μl) of isotonic saline are injected. The pressure in the eye will rise rapidly after this injection but will then soon fall due to normal drainage of fluid.

The peak pressure *after* injection is taken as P_2, and P_1 is the pressure just *prior* to injection. The volume of saline injected is ΔV. As the leveling bulb can be used to change P_1, several pairs of related P_1 and P_2 values may be collected for the same injected volume. An alternative scheme is to inject continuously into the eye starting at a single value of P_1, noting the increase in P_2 as the volume injected increases. Figure 3.6 shows the results for this injection scheme. Figure 3.7 shows a semilog graph of the same data. As these data yield a straight line on the semilog plot, there is a logarithmic increase in pressure with injection of saline.

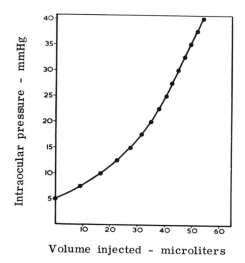

Figure 3.6 Experimentally observed intraocular pressure in the enucleated eye as a functon of the amount injected by means of equipment shown in Figure 3.3. (From Gloster J [1965]: Tonometry and Tonography, Vol. 5, No. 4. International Ophthalmology Clinics. Boston, Little, Brown.)

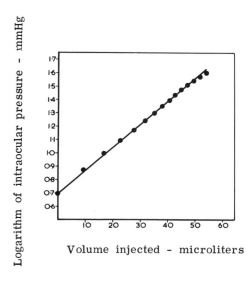

Figure 3.7 Data of Figure 3.6 replotted with logarithm of intraocular pressure on the ordinate. (From Gloster J [1965]: Tonometry and Tonography, Vol. 5, No. 4. International Ophthalmology Clinics. Boston, Little, Brown.)

From the equation of a straight line ($y = ax + b$), Figure 3.7, and rearrangement of Equation 3.7 to $\log P_2 = K \, \Delta V + \log P_1$, it is clear that the intercept on the vertical axis in Figure 3.7 (where ΔV is zero) is $\log P_1$ (here P_1 is 5 mmHg) and the slope of the line through the data points is K, the required ocular rigidity. Ocular rigidity was found to average 0.025 μl^{-1} when measured by this method on several excised human corneas (Gloster 1965).

The effect of using the Schiøtz tonometer may be examined after a value is established for K in the eye under study. The pressure in this eye is set at a value of P_1 by the leveling bulb, and then stopcock T2 is closed. The Schiøtz tonometer is immediately placed on the eye, and the increased pressure (P_2) is measured by the electronic pressure transducer. Since K is known from the previous experiment, Equation 3.6 can be rearranged and used to calculate ΔV:

$$\Delta V = \left(\frac{1}{K}\right) \left(\log \frac{P_2}{P_1}\right) \tag{3.9}$$

The indentation volume of the Schiøtz tonometer may thus be measured for various values of IOP and readings of the tonometer. Essentially, this method compares a pressure change ratio P_2/P_1 due to application of the tonometer to a similar ratio obtained by injecting known volumes of incompressible fluid.

The calibration of the Schiøtz tonometer may now be completed. W is the known weight used on the plunger, and a and b are constants experimentally determined by Friedenwald and Gloster. ΔV for each Schiøtz reading can be read from Figure 3.5. K is taken as 0.025 μl^{-1}. P_1, representing IOP prior to application of the tonometer to the eye, can be calculated for any Schiøtz scale reading R. The chart that accompanies each Schiøtz tonometer (Table 3.2) was constructed by this method; note both pressure and volume of indentation are shown at each reading value.

The volume of indentation for a human eye with an ocular rigidity of 0.025 μl^{-1} and a P_1 of 18 mmHg is about 15 μl. Therefore, the ratio of IOP with the tonometer in place to the IOP without the tonometer on the eye is

$$\frac{P_2}{P_1} = \text{antilog} \, (\Delta V \, K) = \text{antilog} \, (15 \times 0.025) \tag{3.10}$$

Therefore, $P_2/P_1 = 2.37$, or

$$P_2 = 2.37 \, P_1 \tag{3.11}$$

Application of the Schiøtz tonometer to the eye has more than doubled the IOP.

The calibration chart supplied with the Schiøtz tonometer (see Table 3.2) makes the necessary correction to convert instrument readings of P_2 directly to P_1, but it should be noted that this conversion is based on average ocular rigidity and indentation volume values. Although Friedenwald's equation assumes that ocular rigidity is independent of all eye properties and has an average value of 0.025 μl^{-1}, it has been shown to vary in the human population from 0.01 to 0.04 μl^{-1}. This distribution is shown in Figure 3.8 and is from an extensive study of the variation in ocular rigidity in a population of patients from a glaucoma clinic (Gloster 1965);

Table 3.2 Friedenwald's 1955 Calibration for the Schiøtz Tonometer*[+]

	Plunger Weight											
	5.5 gm			7.5 gm			10 gm			15 gm		
Scale Readings	P_1 mmHG	ΔV cu mm	P_2 mmHg	P_1 mmHg	ΔV cu mm	P_2 mmHg	P_1 mmHg	ΔV cu mm	P_2 mmHg	P_1 mmHg	ΔV cu mm	P_2 mmHg
0	41.4	4.4	51.4	59.1	3.4	70.1	81.7	2.7	93.5	127.5	1.9	140.2
0.5	37.8	5.0	48.3	54.2	3.9	65.9	75.1	3.2	87.8	117.9	2.2	131.7
1	34.5	5.6	45.5	49.8	4.5	62.1	69.3	3.6	82.8	109.3	2.6	124.2
1.5	31.6	6.3	43.1	45.8	5.0	58.7	64.0	4.1	78.3	101.4	3.0	117.5
2	29.0	7.0	40.9	42.1	5.7	55.7	59.1	4.6	74.3	94.3	3.4	111.4
2.5	26.6	7.7	38.9	38.8	6.3	53.0	54.7	5.2	70.7	88.0	3.8	106.0
3	24.4	8.5	37.1	35.8	7.0	50.5	50.6	5.8	67.4	81.8	4.3	101.1
3.5	22.4	9.3	35.4	33.0	7.7	48.3	46.9	6.4	64.4	76.2	4.8	96.6
4	20.6	10.1	33.9	30.4	8.5	46.2	43.4	7.1	61.7	71.0	5.3	92.5
4.5	18.9	11.0	32.5	28.0	9.3	44.4	40.2	7.8	59.1	66.2	5.9	88.7
5	17.3	11.9	31.3	25.8	10.1	42.6	37.2	8.6	56.8	61.8	6.5	85.2
5.5	15.9	12.9	30.1	23.8	11.0	41.0	34.4	9.4	54.7	57.6	7.2	82.0
6	14.6	13.9	29.0	21.9	11.9	39.5	31.8	10.2	52.7	53.6	7.8	79.0
6.5	13.4	14.9	28.0	20.1	12.9	38.1	29.4	11.1	50.8	49.9	8.6	76.3
7	12.2	16.0	27.0	18.5	13.9	36.8	27.2	12.0	49.1	46.5	9.3	73.7
7.5	11.2	17.1	26.1	17.0	14.9	35.6	25.1	12.9	47.5	43.2	10.1	71.3
8	10.2	18.3	25.3	15.6	16.0	34.5	23.1	13.9	46.0	40.2	10.9	69.0
8.5	9.4	19.5	24.5	14.3	17.2	33.4	21.3	15.0	44.6	38.1	11.8	66.9
9	8.5	20.7	23.8	13.1	18.3	32.4	19.6	16.0	43.3	34.6	12.7	64.9
9.5	7.8	22.0	23.1	12.0	19.5	31.5	18.0	17.2	42.0	32.0	13.7	63.0
10	7.1	23.3	22.5	10.9	20.8	30.6	16.5	18.3	40.8	29.6	14.7	61.2
10.5	6.5	24.6	21.8	10.0	22.1	29.8	15.1	19.5	39.7	27.4	15.7	59.6
11	5.9	26.0	21.3	9.1	23.4	29.0	13.8	20.8	38.6	25.3	16.8	58.0
11.5	5.3	27.4	20.7	8.3	24.8	28.2	12.6	22.1	37.6	23.3	17.9	56.5
12	4.9	28.8	20.2	7.5	26.2	27.5	11.5	23.4	36.7	21.4	19.1	55.0
12.5	4.4	30.3	19.7	6.8	27.7	26.8	10.5	24.8	35.8	19.7	20.3	53.7
13	4.0	31.9	19.2	6.2	29.2	26.2	9.5	26.2	34.9	18.1	21.5	52.4
13.5		33.4	18.8	5.6	30.7	25.6	8.6	27.7	34.1	16.5	22.8	51.1
14		35.0	18.3	5.0	32.3	25.0	7.8	29.3	33.3	15.1	24.2	50.0
14.5		36.7	17.9	4.5	34.0	24.4	7.1	30.8	32.6	13.7	25.5	48.8
15		38.3	17.5	4.1	35.6	23.9	6.4	32.4	31.9	12.6	27.0	47.8
15.5		40.1	17.1		37.4	23.4	5.8	34.1	31.2	11.4	28.5	46.7
16		41.8	16.8		39.1	22.9	5.2	35.8	30.5	10.4	30.0	45.8
16.5		43.6	16.4		40.9	22.4	4.7	37.6	29.9	9.4	31.5	44.8
17		45.5	16.1		42.8	22.0	4.2	39.4	29.3	8.5	33.2	43.9
17.5		47.3	15.8		44.7	21.5		41.2	28.7	7.7	34.8	43.0
18		49.2	15.5		46.7	21.1		43.1	28.1	6.9	36.5	42.2
18.5		51.2	15.2		48.7	20.7		45.1	27.6	6.2	38.3	41.4
19		53.1	14.9		50.7	20.3		47.1	27.1	5.6	40.1	40.6
19.5		55.2	14.6		52.8	19.9		49.1	26.6	4.9	42.0	39.9
20		57.2	14.4		54.9	19.6		51.2	26.1	4.5	43.9	39.2

*From Friedenwald JS (1957): Tonometer calibration. An attempt to remove discrepancies found in the 1954 Calibration Scale for Schiøtz tonometer. Trans. Am. Acad. Ophthalmol. Otolaryngol. 61:108–123.

[+]Values are given here to one decimal place only. P_1 = pressure in the undisturbed eye; ΔV = volume of corneal indentation; P_2 = intraocular pressure with tonometer resting on the eye.

although most examined eyes were abnormal or diseased in some way, the average value of K is still about 0.025 μl^{-1}. Of the factors that can affect ocular rigidity, special mention should be made of age, IOP itself, and ocular size or volume.

Age tends to increase ocular rigidity; therefore, Schiøtz tonometry measurements could be anticipated to be greater than real IOP with advancing age of the patient examined.

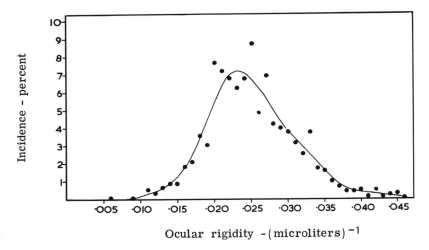

Ocular rigidity -(microliters)$^{-1}$

Figure 3.8 Distribution of ocular rigidity in the human population. (From Gloster J [1965]: Tonometry and Tonography, Vol. 5, No. 4. International Ophthalmology Clinics. Boston, Little, Brown.)

Occasionally the Friedenwald equation is not obeyed, as shown in Figure 3.9, where log P_1 is not linearly related with ΔV; in such an instance ocular rigidity may depend on IOP, as shown in Figure 3.10. Best and his co-workers (1970) have shown that ocular rigidity is highly variable in rabbits; they found K to be a function of both IOP and the size of indentation caused by the Schiøtz tonometer (Figure 3.11).

Ocular rigidity and the calibration of the Schiøtz tonometer are also affected by the volume of the eye. Ocular rigidity is found to be low in myopic eyes with large axial lengths (and subsequently larger volumes), leading to underestimation of true IOP values. The effect of eye volume is intuitively understandable if one considers two spheres of different sizes but identical material. An equal amount of fluid injected into each sphere will cause a greater increase in pressure in the smaller one because there will be a greater fractional increase in volume leading to a greater fractional distention of the sphere's shell. Friedenwald's equation, however, assumes that all eyes have equal volumes and incorporates this "average" volume into the ocular rigidity term (see Equation 3.2). Even if the myopic eye has normal tissue properties, expressed as k in Equation 3.1, Friedenwald's ocular rigidity term K (equal to $k/2.303\ V$) will be low because the tissue property is divided by ocular volume.

If, for example, a value for K of 0.020 μl^{-1}, instead of 0.025 μl^{-1}, had been used in the calculation of P_2/P_1, above (Equation 3.10), this ratio would have been found to be 2.0 instead of 2.37. At a P_1 of 20 mmHg, the difference in the two calculations of P_2 would be 7.4 mmHg. The effect of variation in K is to make the Schiøtz tonometer overestimate IOP in eyes of high ocular rigidity and underestimate IOP in eyes of low ocular rigidity.

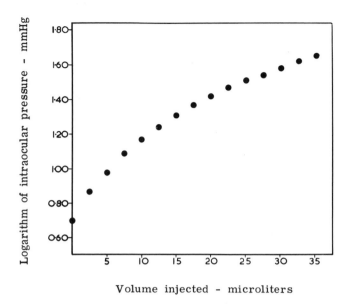

Figure 3.9 Intraocular pressure as a function of volume injected into the eye. This graph shows results sometimes obtained when using the equipment shown in Figure 3.3. The curvature displayed by the experimental points shows that Friedenwald's relationship is not obeyed in this case. (From Gloster J [1965]: Tonometry and Tonography, Vol. 5, No. 4. International Ophthalmology Clinics. Boston, Little, Brown.)

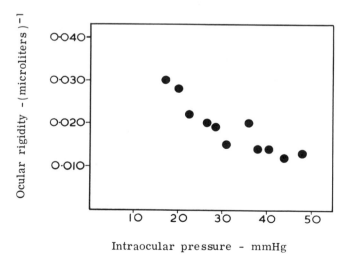

Figure 3.10 Variation of Friedenwald's coefficient of ocular rigidity with intraocular pressure in a human eye. (From Gloster J [1965]: Tonometry and Tonography, Vol. 5, No. 4. International Ophthalmology Clinics. Boston, Little, Brown.)

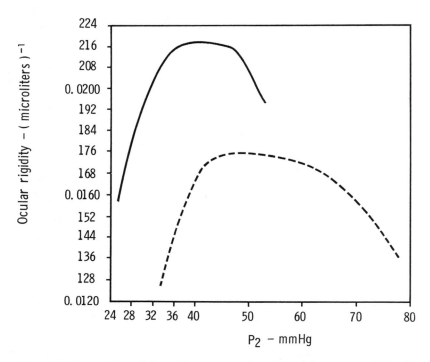

Figure 3.11 Ocular rigidity of the rabbit eye as a function of the pressure P_2 in the eye after the Schiøtz tonometer is applied. The upper curve (———) is for the 5.5-gm weight; the lower curve (----), the10-gm weight. (From Best M, Pola R, Galin MA, Blumenthal M [1970]: Tonometric Calibration for the rabbit eye. Arch. Ophthalmol. 84[2]:200–205. Copyright 1970 American Medical Association.)

McEwen and St. Helen (1965) have suggested that Friedenwald's equation is a simplification of a more general linear relationship

$$\frac{\Delta P}{\Delta V} = aP + b \tag{3.12}$$

where a and b are again constants. When b is zero, Equation 3.12 becomes Friedenwald's equation (Equation 3.6), and the constant a is equivalent to Friedenwald's ocular rigidity K.

Friedenwald suggested the "differential tonometry" method, wherein two separate measurements of IOP are made with two different plunger weights, to avoid the difficulties of using an average ocular rigidity term in the conversion of the Schiøtz scale readings to true IOP. The lower weight (e.g., 5.5 gm) should be used first to minimize the problem of excess drainage of aqueous humor, due to the presence of the weight, contaminating the second measurement. If the 10-gm weight is the second weight, Equation 3.7 can be rewritten for each condition:

$$\log P_1 = \log P_{2(5.5)} - K \, \Delta V_{(5.5)} \tag{3.13}$$

$$\log P_1 = \log P_{2(10)} - K \, \Delta V_{(10)} \tag{3.14}$$

If the two indentation volumes ($\Delta V_{(5.5)}$ and $\Delta V_{(10)}$) are known, and if both true IOP (P_1) and ocular rigidity (K) are considered constant during the two measurements, then Equations 3.13 and 3.14 form a pair of simultaneous equations with the two unknowns K and P_1. The equation for P_1 then eliminates K and becomes

$$\log P_1 = \frac{[\Delta V_{(10)}/\Delta V_{(5.5)}] \log P_{2(5.5)} - \log P_{2(10)}}{[\Delta V_{(10)}/\Delta V_{(5.5)}] - 1} \tag{3.15}$$

Friedenwald recommended that $\Delta V_{(5.5)}$ be taken as 12 µl and $\Delta V_{(10)}$ as 18.5 µl. The terms $P_{2(5.5)}$ and $P_{2(10)}$ are obtained from the Schiøtz scale readings through the use of Equation 3.8 and its average constants.

Although the calculation of P_1 by means of Equation 3.15 seems straightforward, the practical difficulties in obtaining accurate values for $P_{2(5.5)}$ and $P_{2(10)}$ limit the usefulness of differential tonometry. Little accuracy is added by replication of measurements of $P_{2(5.5)}$ and $P_{2(10)}$ because of changes in P_1 during the measurement period. Also, as above, the assumption of a constant K is only an approximation; K can be varied by the increase in pressure caused by the tonometer plunger and added weights. Finally, the use of average $\Delta V_{(5.5)}$ and $\Delta V_{(10)}$ values instead of exact measurements decreases the accuracy of results from Equation 3.15.

Nonetheless, after P_1 is calculated from Equation 3.15, it is possible to use this value in Equation 3.13 or 3.14 to evaluate K. This gives the clinician a means for detecting a value of K that is far from the average.

Despite the limitations of differential tonometry mentioned above, Gloster (1965) points out that the procedure may have some clinical value if it is repeated on one patient during several different clinical examinations. Trends can then be noted, and an approximate value of ocular rigidity defined. This ocular rigidity can then be used during subsequent Schiøtz tonometry measurements on the same patient to improve accuracy in the determination of P_1.

As an alternative to the numerical solution of Equation 3.15, Friedenwald has developed a nomogram from which ocular rigidity can be read directly. Two points representing the two Schiøtz measurements (values of P_2) are located in Figure 3.12 on the Schiøtz scale curves; the line connecting these points is extrapolated to the vertical axis to give the "true" IOP (P_1). A parallel line drawn through the lower left-hand origin of the graph will intercept the protractor curve at the ocular rigidity value.

The practical difficulty in using differential Schiøtz tonometry becomes apparent on examination of the nomogram (Figure 3.12). Small errors in the two tonometry scale readings cause large changes in values for both the slope and intercept of the line connecting the two points that define IOP and ocular rigidity.

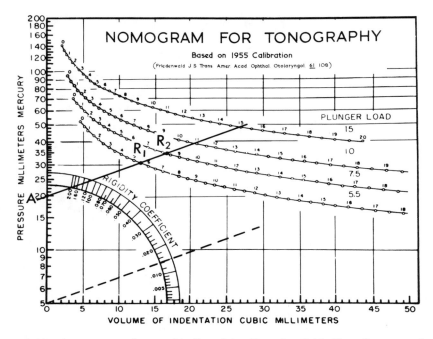

Figure 3.12 A nomogram for graphically solving Equation 3.15. If readings are taken with two different weights, shown as R_1 and R_2, the line connecting R_1 and R_2 can be extrapolated to the vertical axis to give A, the true intraocular pressure. If a parallel line is drawn through the center of the protractor, the ocular rigidity can be read from the protractor scale. (From Gloster J [1965]: Tonometry and Tonography, Vol. 5, No. 4. International Ophthalmology Clinics. Boston, Little, Brown.)

APPLANATION TONOMETRY

Applanation tonometry was developed to decrease the influence of the uncontrolled variables (ocular rigidity and indentation volume) in Schiøtz tonometry. The applanation tonometer developed by Goldmann (and the similar hand-held Clement-Clark Perkins or Kowa versions) measures IOP by observing the force needed to flatten a predetermined area of the corneal surface. The principle of applanation tonometry is shown in Figure 3.13. If the shell of an inflated sphere is infinitely thin, perfectly elastic, and dry, the vertical downward force of the weight W will be balanced by the internal pressure P_1 when the flattened area A is W/P_1 (this is a restatement of the Imbert-Fick law: $W = P_1A$).

The cornea, however, is not infinitely thin, perfectly elastic, nor dry, and therefore the force balance picture is as shown in Figure 3.14. Force s, due to surface tension of the tear film, tends to increase the effective weight, while the finite thickness of the cornea adds a bending force b to the force P_1A caused by the pressure. The relationship between forces is then

$$W + s = P_1A + b \qquad (3.16)$$

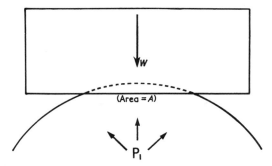

Figure 3.13 Principle of idealized applanation tonometry in which a flat surface block of weight W flattens an area A of the cornea when the intraocular pressure is P_1. (From Gloster J [1965]: Tonometry and Tonography, Vol. 5, No. 4. International Ophthalmology Clinics. Boston, Little, Brown.)

Equation 3.16 can be rearranged to solve for A:

$$A = \left(\frac{W}{P_1}\right) + \left(\frac{s}{P_1}\right) - \left(\frac{b}{P_1}\right) \tag{3.17}$$

When Gloster (1965) tested Equation 3.17 on excised human corneas, he found that the experimental points fell along a line whose equation was

$$A = 63.1 \left(\frac{W}{P_1}\right) + 0.67 \tag{3.18}$$

The term 63.1 is simply a numerical conversion necessary because Gloster expressed W in grams, P_1 in millimeters of mercury, and A in square millimeters. The constant 0.67 is more interesting because it implies that $(s-b)/P_1$ is a constant, that is

$$s - b = 0.67\, P_1 \tag{3.19}$$

This means that the difference between the surface tension force and the bending force is directly proportional to the IOP.

In the absence of surface tension and bending forces, the weight necessary to flatten an area A is given from the definition of pressure, namely

$$W = AP_1 \tag{3.20}$$

since pressure is defined as force (W in a gravitational field g) divided by area. For the units used by Gloster—area in square millimeters, force in grams (weight), and pressure in millimeters of mercury—Equation 3.20 may be rearranged as follows:

$$A = 73.5 \left(\frac{W}{P_1}\right) \tag{3.21}$$

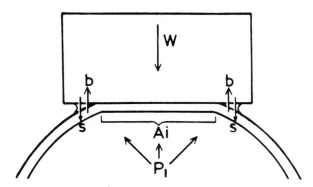

Figure 3.14 Applanation of a cornea by weight W in which the bending of the cornea is resisted by bending force b and enhanced by surface tension force s. (From Gloster J [1965]: Tonometry and Tonography, Vol. 5, No. 4. International Ophthalmology Clinics. Boston, Little, Brown.)

When Gloster plotted both Equations 3.18 and 3.21 on the same graph, he noted that the two lines crossed. He concluded that the surface tension and bending forces were equal and opposite in sign, and therefore cancelled each other at the A and W/P_1 values represented by the crossing point. If the cornea were always flattened to the exact area indicated by this graphical crossing, IOP (or P_1) would be equal to the weight used to flatten the cornea multiplied by a conversion constant.

Gloster first found that the applanation area where bending and surface tension forces cancel was 4.74 mm^2; this is a circle 2.46 mm in diameter. Gloster later found that a more accurate measure of this area was 6.1 mm^2 for human corneas, leading to a corresponding diameter of 2.8 mm. The slightly larger diameter of 3.06 mm was later chosen for the area of applanation to allow direct conversion of grams of force applied to the cornea to millimeters of mercury pressure. For a diameter of 3.06 mm, the circular area is 7.35 mm^2. A force of 1 gm on this area is equivalent to 13.6 gm/cm^2, which is 10 mmHg. Therefore, 1 mmHg IOP is equivalent to 0.1 gm of force on the Goldmann applanation prism, which makes calibration more convenient. If an applanation force is applied to produce a circle of this diameter, there is a simple relation between the force applied and the internal pressure of the eye.

The ability of the Goldmann applanation tonometer to measure IOP with minimum effect of tear surface tension and corneal bending forces does not guarantee that the tonometer is measuring the pressure desired by the clinician. The pressure that is clinically important is that of the undisturbed eye *without* the tonometer in place. The applanation tonometer comes close to giving the pressure of the undisturbed eye because the volume displaced by flattening the cornea to give a 3-mm diameter disk is only 0.54 μl. When this value of ΔV and the average value of K (0.025 μl^{-1}) are substituted into Equation 3.6, the result is

$$\log \left(\frac{P_2}{P_1}\right) = 0.0135 \tag{3.22}$$

Then $P_2/P_1 = 1.032$, or

$$P_1 = 0.969 \, P_2 \tag{3.23}$$

Equation 3.23 shows that the true undisturbed IOP—prior to the application of the applanation tonometer — is about 97% of the tonometer measurement value. This corresponds to an error of about 1 mmHg for normal eyes and 2 mmHg for eyes with abnormally high pressures. Such errors are tolerable in clinical situations.

Note that the effect of ocular rigidity (K) in applanation tonometry is small because K is multiplied by ΔV and ΔV is very small for this kind of tonometry. Applanation tonometry is therefore considered to give IOP measurements independent of ocular rigidity and therefore independent of disease conditions that affect ocular rigidity. The disadvantages of the Goldmann tonometer are that topical anesthesia is still necessary, that the tonometer is expensive compared to the Schiøtz, and that more skill is required to obtain a good measurement with the Goldmann than with the Schiøtz tonometer.

During use of the Goldmann applanation tonometer (Figure 3.15), a transparent plastic plate is forced against the cornea by a spring. This force is controlled by the operator through rotation of a knob with a calibrated scale that indicates the IOP measurement directly in millimeters of mercury. After placing a drop of fluorescein solution on the anesthetized cornea, the applanation plate is brought forward to the corneal surface by using the joystick of the biomicroscope. The operator observes a double semicircular pattern produced by the plate (through one of the microscope oculars) that depends on the diameter of the applanation disk. If the applanation force is too low, the disk is less than 3.06 mm in diameter and the pattern shown in the left-hand side of Figure 3.16 is seen. As the knob is turned to increase the force on the plate, the diameter of contact increases. When the applanating area is exactly 3.06 mm, the pattern shown in the right-hand side of Figure 3.16 is observed and the operator can read the IOP measurement directly off the dial setting.

The Computon microtonometer (CMAT) is a digital electronic tonometer modeled on the Goldmann. This device is hand-held (not mounted on a slitlamp-biomicroscope) and uses internal electronics to monitor the force necessary to flatten a predetermined area of the corneal surface with an applaning titanium membrane.

ERRORS IN TONOMETRY

Gloster (1965) discussed the accuracy of both the Schiøtz and Goldmann tonometers in detail. Apart from the rather obvious requirements that each instrument be properly calibrated, in good working order, and appropriately applied, the most important factor affecting accuracy is the condition of the patient. Apprehension may raise systemic blood pressure and thereby increase the volume

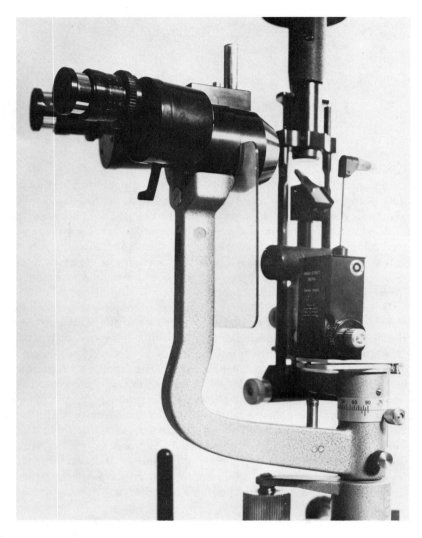

Figure 3.15   The Goldmann tonometer in place on a slitlamp.

of the vascular bed and elevate IOP. Wearing a tight shirt collar or actively holding one's breath may cause venous congestion and thereby raise IOP by increasing the outflow resistance in the episcleral veins. If the eye is inadequately anesthetized, application of either tonometer may cause contraction of the extraocular and lid muscles, which will, by compressing the eye, raise IOP.

From his study of the Schiøtz tonometer, Gloster concluded that the operator's manipulation will lead to errors of about one-half scale division. Another

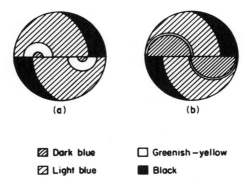

(a)   (b)

▨ Dark blue   ☐ Greenish–yellow
▨ Light blue   ■ Black

Figure 3.16 Patterns seen in the Goldmann tonometer *A*, applanation of required area not yet reached. *B*, correct applanation area. (From Davson H [ed.] [1969]: The Eye, Vol. 1. New York, Academic Press.)

one-half scale division error occurs when observers tend to bias scale readings toward whole division markings. And finally, another one-half scale division error may occur due to variation in the physical properties of the cornea. Since these errors are expected to combine randomly, the overall result is not as bad as one might conclude from this recitation of the possible sources of error. Most Schiøtz readings are within 2 to 5 mmHg of true IOP. Only rarely does a diagnosis need a more accurate measurement of IOP in clinical practice.

The Goldmann applanation tonometer appears to be more accurate than the Schiøtz tonometer. The range of replicate measurements is no more than 2 to 3 mmHg with this tonometer. Problems that may be encountered with use of the Goldmann tonometer are the effects of corneal scars and edema or severe astigmatism. Evidence from studies of animal eyes suggests that corneal properties do affect applanation readings of IOP, but the Goldmann tonometer is a highly accurate device when restricted to human eyes with normal corneas.

A simpler and less expensive type of applanation tonometer is that of Maklakov (Figure 3.17). The version of the Maklakov tonometer available in the United States is called the Tonomat (Figure 3.18). This type of tonometer applies a known force to give a variable area of applanation; this means that tear surface tension and corneal bending force do not necessarily cancel each other.

Gloster's study of the errors in applanation tonometry suggested that ignoring tear surface tension and corneal bending forces would produce readings that are too high. Table 3.3 shows that the error for eyes with IOP in the normal range of 15 to 20 mmHg is tolerable with the 5-gm weight for the Maklakov but becomes greater with heavier weights. For example, a tonometer with the 10-gm weight on an eye with a true IOP of 22 mmHg would measure the IOP as 25 mmHg. This error might tend to induce concern about the health of an eye with a relatively normal true IOP.

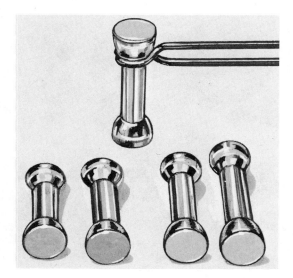

Figure 3.17 The Maklakov tonometer.

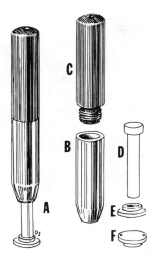

Figure 3.18 The Tonomat tonometer. *A* shows the complete tonometer composed of a hollow barrel (*B*), a solid handle (*C*), plunger (*D*), and applanation plate (*E*). *F* shows the side of the applanation plate that touches the cornea. *D* and *E* together weigh 5.0 gm.

Table 3.3 Errors in Applanation Tonometer When Tear Surface Tension and Corneal Bending Forces Are Ignored

Weight (gm)	IOP Read from Area Measured (mmHg)	True IOP (mmHg)	ΔIOP (mmHg)
5	8.3	7.1	1.1
	12.5	11.1	1.4
	25.0	23.8	1.2
10	16.7	14.3	2.4
	25.0	22.2	2.8
	50.0	47.6	2.4
15	25.0	21.4	3.6
	37.5	33.3	4.2
	75.0	71.4	3.6
20	33.3	28.6	5.7
	50.0	44.4	5.6
	100.0	95.2	4.8

MACKAY-MARG TONOMETER, DURHAM-LANGHAM PNEUMATONOMETERS, AND NONCONTACT TONOMETERS

All previously discussed tonometers require topical corneal anesthesia. The need for a tonometer that could be used without topical anesthetics led to the development of the Mackay-Marg tonometer and Durham-Langham pneuma-tonometer (both of which must touch the eye) and the Grolman-Noncontact tonometer. These are all applanation tonometers because they cause flattening rather than indentation of the cornea. The volume of aqueous humor displaced by corneal flattening is so small that there is little or no effect on ocular rigidity, as discussed earlier.

The mechanical principles of the Mackay-Marg tonometer (introduced in 1959) are shown in Figure 3.19. The operating principle is not exactly the same as in the classical definition of applanation tonometry; although the Mackay-Marg flattens an area of the corneal surface, it does not measure the force to achieve applanation on this entire area. The force required to keep the central plate of a small plunger coplanar with its annular ring is measured instead. This central plunger can move only a few micrometers with respect to the annular guard ring. The force on the plunger is continuously monitored and recorded by a sensitive electronic device. When the tonometer, which is hand-held, is brought to the surface of the cornea, contact is first made with the plunger surface and it

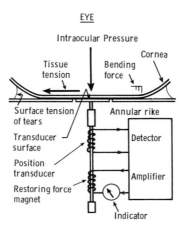

Figure 3.19   Basic parts of the Mackay-Marg tonometer.

is minutely displaced inward from its normal coplanar position. The force required to bring it back to the coplanar position is read out on a chart recorder. As the tonometer is pressed further on the cornea, the flattened area spreads beyond the plunger's central plate and onto the annular guard ring. During this period the force on the plunger decreases and the plunger moves forward toward its original position until the returning force is directly balanced by IOP. Finally, as the operator presses the tonometer even harder against the cornea, IOP itself increases and the plunger records this increase. See Figure 3.20.

The newly introduced Tonopen is similar in operation to the Mackay-Marg tonometer. This device appears to give accurate measurements when the IOP is in the normal range when compared to Goldmann readings, even when used through a bandage soft contact lens (Khan and LaGreca 1989), but it may underestimate Goldmann measurements at high IOPs and overestimate Goldmann measurements at low IOPs (Kao et al. 1987).

The Durham-Langham applanation pneumatonometer has a thin, flexible diaphragm that is pressed against the cornea (Figure 3.21). Inert gas flows through an annular opening behind the diaphragm during operation, but when the anterior surface of the diaphragm is pressed against the ocular surface, its back surface is pushed backward to restrict the gas flow, and the pressure on the diaphragm increases. Gas pressure within the instrument increases until proper applanation is achieved, when gas is again allowed to flow and a whistling sound is produced. A monitoring chart recorder's trace also comes to a wavy plateau (the waves are caused by the patient's pulse); a sample of this is shown in Figure 3.22. The manufacturer claims that the Durham-Langham tonometer will give true IOP readings when applied to the sclera as well as when applied to the cornea. A small downward correction must be made, however, when the sclera is used for measurement. The problem is that the sclera is covered with soft conjunctival and episcleral tissue so that proper applanation is less certain than on the cornea. The

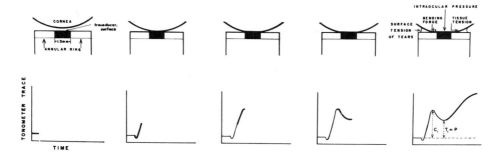

Figure 3.20 The sequence of events as the tonometer probe is advanced toward and on the cornea. Note that as the flattening is increased the trough occurs when the bending forces of the cornea are transferred beyond the sensitive transducer surface to the coplanar surrounding insensitive area or annular ring. C_1, initial crest; T_1, initial trough which yields the intraocular pressure P. Occasionally a tiny initial and final dip from the base line is noted, as shown, because of surface tension attracting the plunger before or after actual contact.

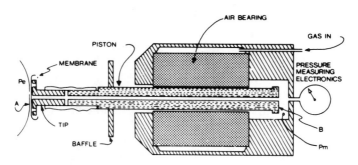

Figure 3.21 Cross-section of the Durham-Langham gas-driven applanation tonometer.

advantage of applying the tonometer to the sclera instead of to the cornea lies in the sclera's lack of sensitivity; the tonometer may then be used without topical anesthesia.

It appears that both the Mackay-Marg and Durham-Langham type of tonometers may give more accurate IOP measurements than does the Goldmann tonometer when used on diseased, scarred, and/or thickened corneas (McMillan and Forster 1975).

The noncontact tonometers (NCT) have been developed more recently. The first was patented by Grolman in 1971 and described a year later (Grolman 1972). The original instrument was from American Optical Company (called the Mk I), but now there are updated Non Contact II and Xpert NCT versions from Reichert as well as several similar devices (one supplied by Keeler, called the Pulsair, another from Topcon, called the CT-20, and also others from both Kowa and Canon).

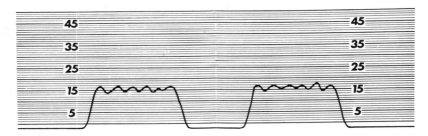

Figure 3.22 Sample record from a Durham-Langham tonometer. The wavy record is caused by the patient's pulse beat. The patient's intraocular pressure is taken as halfway between the peak and trough of the wave. The tonometer paper is imprinted with the intraocular pressure scale. The sample record illustrates an intraocular pressure of 15 mmHg.

These machines produce a puff of air that impinges on the corneal surface to cause applanation. The time interval between the start of the applanation force and the appearance of a flattened cornea is taken as the measure of IOP. The undisturbed cornea is illuminated by light from the source S in Figure 3.23. The observer's task is to focus the optics through the lens system L onto the corneal surface and trigger the pulse of air from the tube T. Note that little of the light reaches the detector after reflection from the undisturbed cornea. On complete applanation of the cornea, all the light from S reaches the detector D_1. Figure 3.24 shows a plot of the applanating force versus time after the puff of air reaches the cornea.

Figure 3.25 combines an oscilloscopic trace showing the development of force on the cornea with the tracing showing output from the light detector. The curve labeled 1 is the record of force applied to the cornea by the air pulse; curve 2 is the applanation spike for an eye with an IOP of 17 mmHg; and curve 3 is the same for an eye with an IOP of 36 mmHg. Note that corneal applanation of a eye with an IOP of 17 mmHg starts about 13 msec after application of the air pulse, whereas an IOP of 36 mmHg slows this time to about 16 msec. The time interval between the start of the applanation force and maximum flattening of the cornea, shown by peak output from the light detector, is counted internally by a crystal-controlled electronic clock. Figure 3.26 shows the relationship between IOP measured on human eyes by Goldmann tonometry and the number of counts of this clock, operated at 10,300 Hz, in NCT measurement.

The NCT converts the number of clock counts, from the start of the air puff to the achievement of corneal flattening, to a measurement of IOP in millimeters of mercury. Figure 3.27 shows the relationship between Goldmann and NCT measurements in millimeters of mercury after this conversion is made.

The NCT appears to be an important advance in clinical tonometry because the device makes no direct contact with the eye being measured, thereby eliminating the need for anesthesia or sterilization procedures. A minimum amount of operator skill or judgment is needed. At present, however, disadvantages include

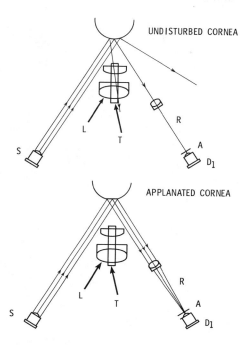

Figure 3.23 Schematic diagram of the optical system in Grolman's noncontact tonometer. Light originates at light source *S*, strikes cornea and is reflected to telescope *R* and then through aperture *A* to light detector D_1. The orientation of the cornea is observed through the optical system *L*. The air puff is directed to the cornea via tube *T*. In the upper figure, the cornea has not yet been applanated; thus, very little reflected light is being returned to the detector D_1. In the lower figure, the applanated cornea reflects all or most of the light to the detector. (From Grolman B [1972]: A new tonometer system. Am J. Optom. 49:646–660.)

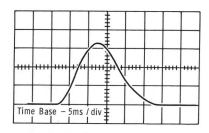

AIR PULSE FORCE–TIME ENVELOPE — AS
SENSED BY FORCE TRANSDUCER LOCATED
AT 11 mm. FROM ORIFICE OF TUBE T

Figure 3.24 Force of an air puff as a function of time as sensed by a force transducer 11 mm in front of the orifice. This force diagram is representative of the force applied to the cornea.

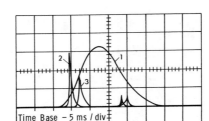

Figure 3.25 Combined force-time trace, as shown in Figure 3.24, with the output of the light detector D_1. (From Grolman B [1972]: A new tonometer system. Am. J. Optom. 49:646–660.)

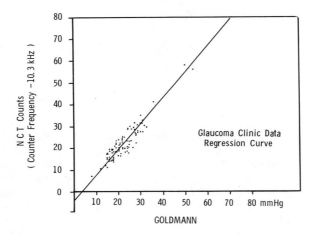

Figure 3.26 Correlation between Goldmann tonometer readings and NCT counts (equivalent to time for applanation) when both measurements are made on the same human subjects. (From Grolman B [1972]: A new tonometer system. Am. J. Optom. 49:646–660.)

cost, the sound of the air puff (which can be disturbing to the patient), and the unavailability of a calibrating device to be used by the practitioner to check accuracy from time to time. Forbes and colleagues (1974) also found that the NCT might not be the most accurate tonometer to use on eyes with edematous corneas or low visual acuities.

Sorensen (1975) made the following observations after a well-designed statistical study of NCT results:

1. If the patient can quickly fixate (in less than 3 seconds), the average of several NCT measurements may be more accurate than just the first measurement because repeated exposures to the NCT do not raise IOP.

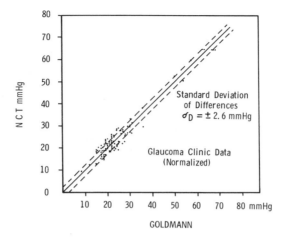

Figure 3.27 Data of Figure 3.26 replotted to shift the least squares fitted line to the origin. The ordinate has been converted to millimeters of mercury. (From Grolman B [1972]: A new tonometer system. Am. J. Optom. 49:646–660.)

2. Good fixation is essential. There is increased error in NCT measurements when amblyopes and eccentric fixators are examined.
3. NCT readings correlate very well with Goldmann tonometry measurements when the cornea is clear and IOP is less than 35 mmHg; at IOP values above 45 mmHg the NCT begins to lose precision.
4. A grossly diseased (scarred, edematous, or irregularly surfaced) cornea leads to unreliable NCT readings.

In a 1990 study of all commercially available air-puff tonometers, Brencher and co-workers (1991) concluded that they are useful clinical tools but must be used with caution. In the normal range of IOPs these tonometers are of value for screening purposes. When there is suspicion of a pressure outside the normal range, follow-up testing with a Goldmann tonometer is required.

THE NORMAL INTRAOCULAR PRESSURE

Leydhecker and co-workers (1958) studied IOP by Schiøtz tonometry in 13,861 healthy subjects. Their results are shown graphically in Figure 3.28. The mode (most common) pressure was found to be approximately 16 mmHg; about 35% of the population studied had this pressure, and the pressures in 95% of the eyes tested were in the range of 10.5 to 20.5 mmHg. Clinically, a pressure above 20.5 mmHg is abnormal, and one greater than 25 mmHg is definitely pathological.

Applanation tonometry gives a mean population value of 15.4 (SD ± 2.5) mmHg for sitting patients and 16.5 (SD ± 2.6) mmHg for reclining patients. Care

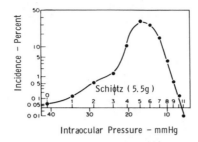

Figure 3.28 Distribution of intraocular pressure in the human population. Measurements were made with the Schiøtz tonometer. Note logarithmic scale for incidence. (From Davson H [ed.] [1969]: The Eye, Vol. 1. New York, Academic Press.)

must be exercised when interpreting these statistics, since the distributions are skewed, as shown in Figure 3.28.

The differences between indentation and applanation tonometry tend to decrease when large populations are studied. Table 3.4 shows the results of nine studies; the mean values for IOP by indentation (Schiøtz) and applanation (Goldmann) tonometry are essentially the same, and other statistical measures are almost identical as well.

Table 3.4 Intraocular Pressure (in mmHg) in Normal Human Subjects from Nine Studies as Indicated*

Study	Impression Tonometry (Schiøtz)			Applanation Tonometry (Goldmann)		
	M	SD	M + 3 SD	M	SD	M + 3 SD
Goldmann and Schmidt 1957	15.5	2.80	M + 3	14.45	2.50	M + 3
Goldmann and Schmidt 1957	—	—	—	15.45	2.52	23.0
Leydhecker, Akiyama, and Neumann 1958	15.5	2.57	23.2	—	—	—
Becker 1958	16.1	2.80	24.5	—	—	—
Linnér 1958	15.2	2.47	22.6	—	—	—
Draeger 1959	—	—	—	14.5	2.80	22.9
Weekers et al. 1959	—	—	—	16.3	2.50	23.8
Kruse 1960	13.5	2.61	21.3	13.7	2.50	21.2
Saeteren 1960	14.3	1.91	20.0	14.0	1.74	19.2
Graham and Hollows 1964	15.1	2.90	23.8	16.3	3.00	25.3

M = mean; SD = standard deviation.

*From Gloster J (1965): Tonometry and Tonography, Vol. 5, No. 4. International Ophthalmology Clinics. Boston, Little, Brown.

Values of IOP in the lower animals may be of interest. The best value for the rabbit is probably 17.6 mmHg, measured by direct tap of the posterior chamber without general anesthesia. Davson (1969) found a mean value of 16.5 mmHg (range of 7.5 to 22 mmHg) for the IOP of the anesthetized cat. The IOP of monkeys is definitely lower, always about 12 mmHg, but varies with exact species.

FACTORS AFFECTING THE INTRAOCULAR PRESSURE

Age itself appears to have little effect on IOP. Costagliola and associates (1990) observed only a slight, and insignificant, increase in IOP with age (from 15 to 17 mmHg) as measured by Goldmann tonometry in 751 subjects (1502 eyes) in an urban area in Italy. Age was over the range of 6 to 89 years. Half of this increase (i.e., 1 mmHg) was noted over the first 60 years of age, and the other half between ages 61 to 70 and 81 to 89. This is consistent with the study of McLeod and co-workers (1990) who, using data from electronic Schiøtz measurements of 572 male subjects (age 25 to 85 years) studied during the Baltimore Longitudinal Study on Aging, found that changes in IOP over time are associated with changes in systolic blood pressure and that IOP does not necessarily increase with age. As ocular rigidity tends to increase with age, however, there is a tendency for measurements taken with the Schiøtz tonometer to be higher for more aged individuals unless a correction is made for the increased value of K.

IOP varies with time of day. It appears to be highest early in the morning and lowest in the evening. The variation is about 4 mmHg. Ericson (1958) claimed that changes in the rate of aqueous humor secretion are responsible. Another causative factor, however, for this variation could be changes in the muscular activities of the ciliary muscle and/or iris due to light. Diurnal variations should be interpreted with great care since some normal subjects may have a reversed diurnal variation. Of interest, the glaucomatous patient may have a much higher diurnal variation (8 to 10 mmHg) than does the nonglaucomatous patient, and the maximum pressure may occur at any time of the day or night. Kitazawa and Horie (1975) found that IOP fell to a normal level at some time during the day in at least half of their open-angle glaucoma patients. This finding demonstrates the need for repeated IOP measurements at various times of day for any patient suspected of having glaucoma.

Systemic blood pressure appears to have little acute effect on the IOP of normal eyes. A transient rise in blood pressure is followed by a small, transient rise in IOP—but usually only about 10% of the rise in blood pressure (Duke-Elder 1968). There is no consistent relationship between chronic vascular hypertension and IOP in normal eyes.

Daubs (1976), however, indicates that the ratio of blood pressure to IOP is shifted down in glaucomatous patients. Figure 3.29 shows his results in a frequency distribution of systolic blood pressure/IOP ratios for a group of 243 patient measurements (where about half the patients had a diagnosis of glaucoma).

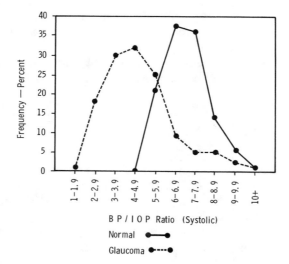

Figure 3.29 Frequency distribution of blood pressure/IOP ratios in normal and glaucomatous patients. (From Daubs J [1976]: A retrospective analysis of the systolic BP/IOP ratio in glaucoma screening. J. Am. Optom. Assoc. 47:450–455. (Reprinted with permission of the Journal of the American Optometric Association.)

Although systemic blood pressure has little direct effect on IOP itself, it may participate in the expression of glaucoma. Nerve damage in this disease may occur from direct pressure on the ocular blood supply; high IOP may cause visual damage by "pinching off" some of the small capillaries supplying the nerve fibers. Increasing systemic blood pressure may have a small role in preventing increased IOP from reducing the perfusion of these small vessels. On the other hand, reduction in systemic blood pressure might reduce blood flow and perfusion to the retina, thereby increasing the potential for field loss at a lower IOP (Kolker and Hetherington 1983). This is not the only mechanism, however, proposed to explain the loss of vision in glaucoma; one alternative is that increased IOP directly compresses or bends the optic nerve itself where it leaves the eye at the lamina cribrosa.

A model of liquid flow paths in the eye will aid in understanding the influence of various physiological factors on IOP. Figure 3.30 shows the flow paths and pressures diagrammatically. The aqueous humor is produced from arterial blood flowing at pressure P_{ia} through the arteries of the ciliary body. As metabolic work is required to move fluid from the arteries to the inside chambers of the eye, the location where such work is performed is a *pump* in the ciliary epithelium. Fluid leaves the eye through the trabecular meshwork and canal of Schlemm and by percolation through the uveoscleral tract. The flow of fluid through both the canal of Schlemm and uveoscleral route is related to the pressure drop across these

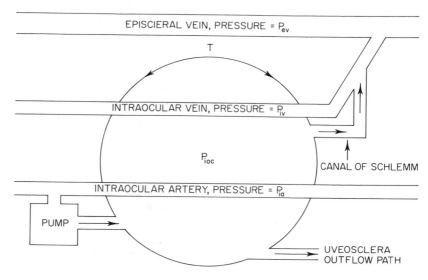

Figure 3.30 Liquid flow paths in the eye. (From Davson H [ed.] [1969]: The Eye, Vol. 1. New York, Academic Press.)

outflow paths just as the flow of electricity through a resistor is related to a voltage drop in Ohm's law. For the canal of Schlemm, we can write

$$P_{ioc} - P_{ev} = R_c F_c \qquad (3.24)$$

where P_{ioc} is the pressure inside the eye, P_{ev} is the pressure in the episcleral veins into which the aqueous humor is discharged, R_c is the flow resistance in the canal of Schlemm (considered mainly at the inner wall of the canal or in the trabecular meshwork adjacent to the canal), and F_c is the flow rate through this pathway. For the uveoscleral tract, we can write

$$P_{ioc} = R_u F_u \qquad (3.25)$$

where R_u is the resistance and F_u is the flow rate through the uveoscleral tract. No term equivalent to P_{ev} exists here because we are uncertain where the fluid goes; if it goes into the orbit or conjunctival sac the pressure there is zero and so the driving force is then simply P_{ioc}.

The sum $F_c + F_u$ must be equal to F_o (the drainage rate of aqueous humor from the eye). As inflow must equal outflow in the eye, however, the production rate F must equal the absolute value of outflow:

$$F = F_o = F_c + F_u \qquad (3.26)$$

If we combine Equations 3.24, 3.25, and 3.26 and solve for P_{ioc}, we obtain

$$P_{ioc} = \frac{(R_c F + P_{ev})}{(1 + \{R_c/R_u\})} \qquad (3.27)$$

The pressure developed in the eye inflates this sphere until the tension induced in the shell balances the inflation pressure. The tension (T) in the shell is given by

$$T = \frac{(P_{ioc}r)}{2} \tag{3.28}$$

where r is the shell radius. Inserting the solution for P_{ioc} from Equation 3.27 into Equation 3.28 and rearranging gives

$$T = \left(\frac{r}{2}\right) \left(\frac{[R_c F + P_{ev}]}{[1 + \{R_c/R_u\}]} \right) \tag{3.29}$$

Equation 3.29 shows how the tension in the ocular shell is related to the aqueous humor production rate, episcleral venous pressure, and the resistances to outflow. Equations 3.27 and 3.29 are also, however, based on the assumption that each term on the right-hand side of these equations is independent of the other terms. When a human patient experiences an attack of "angle-closure" glaucoma, the iris collapses on the posterior peripheral corneal surface and the resistance to outflow of aqueous humor through the canal of Schlemm increases. IOP may rise as high as 60 to 80 mmHg, in the direction predicted by Equations 3.27 and 3.29, although there is still no assurance that F and P_{ev} have remained constant. If changes do occur, such differences are obviously not enough to counter the effect of increasing R_c.

Blood flowing into the vascular system of the eye is at the pressure of the body's arterial system. The ocular arteries, however, have relatively thick walls of low extensibility. Most of the arterial pressure is therefore taken up as tension in these arterial walls, and very little is available to influence IOP. Arterial pulsations appear as a superimposed pressure variation on the relatively constant IOP; Figure 3.31 shows a record of IOP from the eye of an anesthetized living rabbit as observed with an ocular tap connecting the globe to an electronic pressure transducer (see Figure 3.3). There is a 1 second/cycle pressure pulse due to breathing, and superimposed on this is the pulse corresponding to cardiac systole and diastole. Although the peak-to-trough difference in height of the arterial pressure graph is about 20 mmHg, the damping effect of the arterial walls reduces the ocular pulse to only about 1 mmHg.

When IOP increases while arterial pressure is held constant, there is an accompanying decrease in the pressure difference across the arterial wall. This causes a reduction in the stretching tension in this wall, and the vessel increases its pulsation amplitude. Further increase in IOP, however, will collapse the artery, and the pulsations will disappear. This explains the clinical observation of the initial increase and subsequent decrease in pulsation of the ocular blood vessels as IOP increases.

Venous pulsation is commonly noted during ophthalmoscopic examination of the optic disk in normal eyes; pressure in this vein can apparently vary above and below IOP. The blood pressure in the episcleral veins (see P_{iv} in Figure 3.30), however, must be above IOP at all times or these vessels would collapse and close the aqueous humor outflow path or allow for fluid (perhaps blood) backflow.

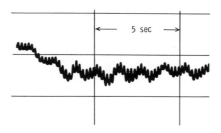

Figure 3.31 Record from the pressure transducer shown in Figure 3.3 when connected directly to the anterior chamber of a living, anesthetized rabbit.

Episcleral venous pressure (P_{ev} in Figure 3.30) is at the low venous pressure of the large venous trunks (10 to 14 mmHg), so there must be a sudden drop in pressure in the veins as they pass from the eye into the soft episcleral tissue. Several authors (Baurmann 1925; Swann 1954; Davson 1956) suggest that a sudden drop of pressure along a vein is a condition that will favor pulsatile flow.

ESTIMATING CHANGES IN INTRAOCULAR PRESSURE

An increase in pressure in the intraocular veins has two separate effects on IOP. First, when the pressure inside the thin-walled retinal and choroidal veins is suddenly increased, there is an increase in the vein diameter because the walls have little resistance to distention. This increase in vein volume is equivalent to a decrease in intraocular volume and will cause a sudden rise in IOP, as predicted by Friedenwald's equation. However, the extra internal pressure will soon disappear as an equivalent volume of aqueous humor drains out of the eye to restore the original pressure.

The second, and long-term, effect of increasing venous pressure is clear from an examination of Equation 3.27 rearranged to

$$P_{ioc} = \left[\frac{(R_c F)}{(1 + R_c/R_u)} \right] + \left[\frac{P_{ev}}{(1 + R_c/R_u)} \right] \tag{3.30}$$

If we still assume that outflow is divided 80% via Schlemm's canal and 20% via the uveoscleral tract (see Chapter 2), then $1 + R_c/R_u$ is 1.056. If both this relationship and the production rate of aqueous humor (F) are constant, the differentiation of Equation 3.30 gives

$$dP_{ioc} = 0 + \left(\frac{1}{1.056} \right) dP_{ev} = 0.95 \, dP_{ev} \tag{3.31}$$

This indicates that a change in episcleral venous pressure will cause an almost equivalent change in IOP.

An estimate of the effect of change in aqueous humor production rate on IOP can also easily be made from Equation 3.30 if outflow via the uveoscleral tract is ignored for the moment. By this assumption, R_c/R_u is zero as R_u is infinite, and Equation 3.30 becomes

$$P_{ioc} = R_c F + P_{ev} \tag{3.32}$$

Assuming P_{ev} is constant, differentiation gives

$$dP_{ioc} = R_c \, dF \tag{3.33}$$

But, $R_c = (P_{ioc} - P_{ev})/F$ by rearrangement of Equation 3.24. Substituting this for R_c in Equation 3.33 and dividing both sides by P_{ioc} gives

$$\frac{dP_{ioc}}{P_{ioc}} = \left(1 - \frac{P_{ev}}{P_{ioc}}\right) \frac{dF}{F} \tag{3.34}$$

If we take P_{ioc} as 18 mmHg (a normal value) and P_{ev} as 10 mmHg (as experimentally observed), then the term $(1 - P_{ev}/P_{ioc})$ is 0.44 and

$$\frac{dP_{ioc}}{P_{ioc}} = 0.44 \frac{dF}{F} \tag{3.35}$$

Equation 3.35 shows that the fractional change in IOP will be only 44% of the fractional change in aqueous flow rate if the uveoscleral tract is ignored.

To include the uveoscleral outflow in this calculation, one must start from the previously determined relationship for total outflow, Equation 3.26: $F_o = F_c + F_u$. Substituting rearrangements of Equations 3.24 and 3.25 from above gives us

$$F_o = \left[\frac{(P_{ioc} - P_{ev})}{R_c}\right] + \left[\frac{P_{ioc}}{R_u}\right] \tag{3.36}$$

Solving Equation 3.36 for P_{ioc}

$$P_{ioc} = \frac{(F_o R_c R_u + R_u P_{ev})}{(R_c + R_u)} \tag{3.37}$$

or, as $F_o = F$, by rearrangement

$$P_{ioc} = F\left[\frac{R_c R_u}{(R_c + R_u)}\right] + \left[\frac{R_u P_{ev}}{(R_c + R_u)}\right] \tag{3.38}$$

Differentiating Equation 3.38, while assuming P_{ev} is constant, yields

$$dP_{ioc} = \left[\frac{R_c R_u}{(R_c + R_u)}\right] dF \tag{3.39}$$

Dividing Equation 3.39 by Equation 3.37, and reducing to its simplest form, gives

$$\frac{dP_{ioc}}{P_{ioc}} = \left[\frac{1}{(1 + \{P_{ev}/FR_c\})}\right] \frac{dF}{F} \tag{3.40}$$

Additionally, when both sides of Equation 3.36 are multiplied by R_c, it becomes

$$FR_c = (P_{ioc} - P_{ev}) + P_{ioc} \left(\frac{R_c}{R_u}\right) \tag{3.41}$$

and using values of 18 mmHg for P_{ioc} and 10 mmHg for P_{ev}, as previously assumed, and where $R_c/R_u = 0.056$ as previously determined, Equation 3.41 becomes

$$FR_c = 9.01 \text{ mmHg} \tag{3.42}$$

This number may now be used in Equation 3.40, and with P_{ev} still equal to 10 mmHg, we find

$$\frac{dP_{ioc}}{P_{ioc}} = 0.47 \frac{dF}{F} \tag{3.43}$$

Equation 3.43 shows that the fractional change in IOP is 47% of the fractional change in aqueous humor production when uveoscleral outflow is considered in addition to the more conventional route.

The effect of changes in episcleral venous pressure on IOP might also be of interest. Differentiation of Equation 3.38, after assuming that $F[R_cR_u/(R_c + R_u)]$ is a constant, gives

$$dP_{ioc} = \left[\frac{R_u}{(R_c + R_u)} \right] dP_{ev} \tag{3.44}$$

If it is again assumed that 80% of outflow is along Schlemm's canal and 20% by the uveoscleral route, then

$$dP_{ioc} = 0.95 \, dP_{ev} \tag{3.45}$$

Note that differentiation of Equation 3.32 with the uveoscleral pathway ignored and with R_cF held constant would predict that $dP_{ioc} = dP_{ev}$. It is therefore clear that a change in the episcleral venous pressure is reflected as almost an identical change in IOP, whether or not the uveoscleral route is considered.

FACILITY OF OUTFLOW AND TONOGRAPHY

Although evaluation of Equations 3.24 and 3.38 with numerical values on the right-hand side of each equation would lead one to the belief that FR_c and $F[R_cR_u/(R_c + R_u)]$ are less important than either P_{ev} or $P_{ev}R_u/(R_c + R_u)$ in the control of IOP, this is clinically not the case. Both F and R_c can be greatly changed by pathological processes inside the eye, thereby causing P_{ioc} to increase substantially, with potentially vision-threatening consequences, while P_{ev} remains relatively stable.

Since it is the products FR_c or $F[R_c/(1 + \{R_c/R_u\})]$ that will cause P_{ioc} to increase, one should measure either F or R_c (assuming that the ratio R_c/R_u is close to 1) when IOP is elevated, to determine which factor is responsible. The aqueous flow rate F is difficult to measure except with tracers, and even then the procedure is not suitable for clinical use. Therefore, the determination of R_c becomes the measurement of choice. If R_c is normal, then the increase in P_{ioc} must be due to changes in F by process of elimination.

When P_{ev} is considered constant and Equation 3.36 is differentiated, the result is

$$\frac{dF}{dP_{ioc}} = \frac{[R_c + R_u]}{R_c R_u} = \frac{[(R_c/R_u) + 1]}{R_c} \quad (3.46)$$

If the outflow via the uveoscleral pathway is ignored (i.e., $R_u = \infty$) to simplify this concept, then

$$\frac{dF}{dP_{ioc}} = \frac{1}{R_c} \quad (3.47)$$

The terms on the right-hand sides of Equations 3.46 and 3.47 are given the symbol C in the ophthalmological literature, and either is called the *facility of outflow*, or simply the *facility*. Equations 3.46 and 3.47 show clearly that C is the inverse of resistance and could alternatively be called the "outflow conductance," as these equations are the fluid-flow analogs of Ohm's law in electricity: F is equivalent to current, and P_{ioc} is equivalent to voltage.

Consideration of Equations 3.46 and 3.47 indicates that the relationship between aqueous humor flow rate and IOP will be linear and the slope of this relationship will be C, provided episcleral venous pressure is constant. The process of increasing IOP by placing a tonometer on an eye and then observing the gradual induced fall in pressure as this weight promotes increased aqueous humor drainage is called *tonography*. Tonographic measurements therefore yield data from which the facility can be calculated. A tonograph is simply a Schiøtz tonometer modified to give a continuous electrical recording of its scale reading. The Mueller tonograph is a commercial version of such a device.

Ophthalmic clinicians infrequently perform tonography, but the mechanisms that control IOP can be better understood after a discussion of the principles of the tonographic procedure. Gloster's (1965) explanation of the various pressure changes during tonography will be given here. The uveoscleral pathway is ignored, but the error introduced by this is not important.

Consistent with the analogy to Ohm's law made earlier, the aqueous humor outflow rate via Schlemm's canal prior to placement of the tonographic instrument on the cornea (F_c) is related to IOP by a rearrangement of Equation 3.24, where $C = 1/R_c$:

$$F_c = C (P_{ioc} - P_{ev}) \quad (3.48)$$

P_{ioc} is instantaneously increased when the tonometer is placed on the cornea due to the indentation produced by the Schiøtz-type tonometer because there is insufficient time for all the displaced aqueous humor to exit via the outflow channel. The extra pressure thus generated stretches the tunic of the eye, mostly the sclera. There is, of course, also an immediate increase in the rate of outflow due to increased IOP. Let us assume that the new higher IOP is P' and it remains at this value. The increase in IOP will increase the outflow from F_c to F_c', where $F_c' = F_c + f$, and f is the increase in flow rate due to the increase in IOP on applying the tonometer. Based on Equation 3.48, the new flow rate $(F_c + f)$ must be related to the facility of outflow (C) through

$$F_c + f = C\,(P' - P_{ev}) \tag{3.49}$$

Equation 3.49 is not quite correct because we know from other experiments that the presence of such an instrument on the cornea also raises P_{ev} by an amount ΔP_{ev}. The aqueous humor flowing out of the eye via Schlemm's canal therefore encounters the increased pressure $P_{ev} + \Delta P_{ev}$, and Equation 3.49 becomes

$$F_c + f = C\,[P' - (P_{ev} + \Delta P_{ev})] \tag{3.50}$$

When Equations 3.48 and 3.50 are solved for F_c and the two resulting equations set equal to each other, we obtain

$$C = \frac{f}{(P' - P_{ioc} - \Delta P_{ev})} \tag{3.51}$$

Equation 3.51 becomes the basis of the calculation of facility of outflow, C, in tonography.

The increase in aqueous humor outflow may also be written

$$f = \frac{\Delta V}{t} \tag{3.52}$$

where ΔV is the extra volume of the aqueous outflow during time t of the application of the tonograph instrument. Inserting Equation 3.52 into Equation 3.51

$$C = \frac{\Delta V}{[t(P' - P_{ioc} - P_{ev})]} \tag{3.53}$$

Equation 3.53 was derived assuming that IOP increases to P' by application of the tonograph and then remains at this elevated pressure for the full period t. This is of course not the case. Since the tonograph instrument is usually held on the eye for 4 minutes, the subscript "4" will be used to indicate a property of the system at the end of this duration. Similarly, the subscript "o" will indicate the same property at the beginning of the 4-minute application period, at an instant in time just after the instrument is placed on the eye. Application of the tonograph raises IOP to P' only momentarily; and then P' begins to fall. The usual practice in tonography is to take P' as the average value during the 4-minute period; P_o is the initial pressure just after the instrument is applied to the eye, and P_4 is the final pressure at the 4-minute mark. Thus,

$$P' = \frac{(P_o + P_4)}{2} \tag{3.54}$$

The equation for facility of outflow becomes

$$C = \frac{\Delta V}{t[\{(P_o + P_4)/2\} - P_{ioc} - \Delta P_{ev}]} \tag{3.55}$$

Figure 3.32 shows the eye before application of the tonographic instrument in the left-hand figure; the indentation and increased IOP immediately after application in the center figure; and the increased indentation and reduced IOP after 4 minutes in the right-hand figure. The volume changes in the eye are shown in more detail in Figure 3.33. The extra volume of fluid ΔV that is displaced from the eye during the 4-minute application period can be treated as being the sum of two components. There is first a corneal component (ΔV_c) caused by the slow sinking of the tonographic plunger into the cornea as pressure falls from the instantaneous high value immediately after application of the instrument. The second part is ΔV_s, the change in volume due to the decrease in scleral extension as IOP falls from its highest value at time t_o. Therefore, $\Delta V = \Delta V_c + \Delta V_s$. The scleral portion ($\Delta V_s$) can be evaluated from Friedenwald's equation: $\log P_1/P_2 = K\Delta V_s$. Therefore, $\Delta V = \Delta V_c + (1/K) [\log P_o - \log P_4]$, and this value may be substituted into Equation 3.55 to give a new equation for the facility of outflow:

$$C = \frac{V_c + (1/K) [\log P_o - \log P_4]}{t[(P_o + P_4)/2 - P_{ioc} - \Delta P_{ev}]} \quad (3.56)$$

All the terms in Equation 3.56 can be obtained from the tonographic measurements or from the tables available in the text by Drews (1971). The term t is

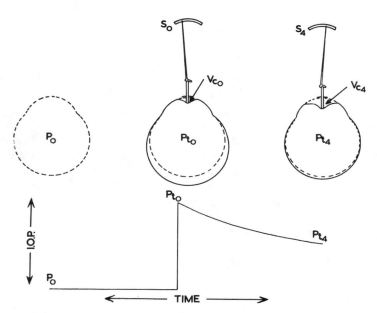

Figure 3.32 Changes in volume and pressure of the eye during tonography. (From Gloster J [1965]: Tonometry and Tonography, Vol. 5, No. 4. International Ophthalmology Clinics. Boston, Little, Brown.)

the time the tonographic instrument is held on the eye, usually 4 minutes. ΔV_c is the difference in corneal indentations at pressures P_4 and P_o. These two pressures are taken from the respective Schiøtz readings using the values given in Table 3.2. Table 3.2 also provides corneal indentations for each reading. The ocular rigidity can be taken as the average value for the human population described above: 0.025 μl^{-1}. The value of ΔP_{ev} may be taken as 1.25 mmHg from the experimental work of Linnér (1958).

The use of an average value for ocular rigidity is a potentially serious problem with Equation 3.56 because there is no allowance for an individual ocular variation in this parameter. Equation 3.56 is therefore said to give an "uncorrected" facility of outflow.

An alternative procedure is available to obtain facility of outflow without assuming an average ocular rigidity value. This method requires the use of an applanation tonometer in conjunction with the normal tonograph. The facility of outflow thus measured is then the "corrected facility." In practice, this procedure is very much simplified by use of a nomogram (Figure 3.34).

Figure 3.35 shows a typical tonographic record. This patient has an applanation IOP measurement of 17 mmHg; this is shown in Figure 3.34 by an X at this location on the left-hand vertical axis. When the tonographic instrument, an electronic Schiøtz gauge, is placed on the eye with the 5.5-gm weight, the initial reading obtained is 4.0, shown as point Q on Figure 3.34; this represents a pressure of 34 mmHg as shown by drawing a horizontal line from point Q to its interception of the vertical axis. After 4 minutes, the plunger has sunk into the cornea and the Schiøtz reading is 7.0 (shown as R), and a horizontal line from R to its interception of the vertical axis of the graph shows that IOP has decreased to 27 mmHg. Vertical lines dropped from Q and R to the horizontal axis of the nomogram indicate that corneal indentation initially displaced 10 μl and increased to 16 μl by the end of the 4-minute measurement period. ΔV_c is thereby 16 − 10 μl, or 6 μl.

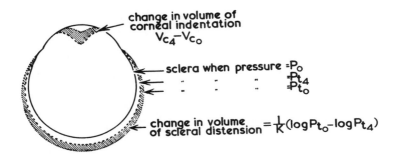

Figure 3.33 Details of volume change of the eye during tonography. (From Gloster J [1965]: Tonometry and Tonography, Vol. 5, No. 4. International Ophthalmology Clinics. Boston, Little, Brown.)

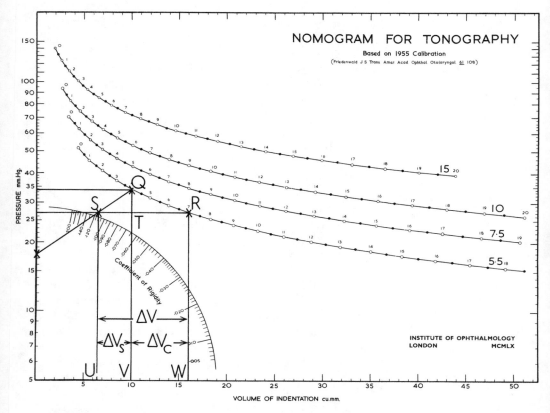

Figure 3.34 Nomogram for calculating the facility of outflow from tonograph data. (Reprinted with permission of Institute of Ophthalmology, London.)

The slope of the line connecting point X to point Q is given by

$$\text{Slope} = \frac{QT}{ST} \qquad (3.57)$$

but, as the vertical axis of this graph is logarithmic, it is also true that

$$QT = \log P_o - \log P_4 \qquad (3.58)$$

From Friedenwald's equation (3.6)

$$\Delta V_s = \frac{(\log P_o - \log P_4)}{K} \qquad (3.59)$$

Therefore

$$\Delta V_s = \frac{QT}{K} \qquad (3.60)$$

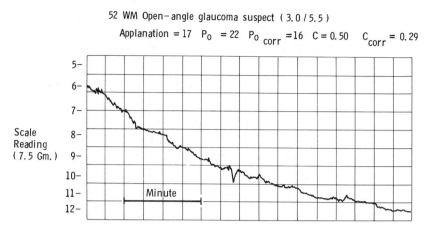

Figure 3.35 Tonograph record from a 52-year-old white male patient suspected of having open-angle glaucoma. From Kolker AE, Hetherington J Jr [1970]: Becker-Schaffer's diagnosis and Therapy of the Glaucomas, ed. 3. St. Louis, C.V. Mosby.

The nomogram has been constructed as a semilogarithmic graph so that the slope QT/ST also represents ocular rigidity K, and therefore

$$\Delta V_s = \frac{QT}{(QT/ST)} = ST \tag{3.61}$$

The distance ST carried down to the horizontal axis of the graph gives ΔV_s, which is 3.5 µl in Figure 3.34. The total extra outflow of fluid thereby is $6 + 3.5 = 9.5$ µl. In practice, the line from Q to the vertical axis need not be drawn since vertical lines from S and R will give the total ΔV.

This total displaced volume divided by 4 minutes gives 2.375 µl/min. The average pressure during this time period was $(34 + 27)/2 = 30.5$ mmHg, as read from the horizontal lines drawn from Q and R to the vertical axis in Figure 3.34. Normal IOP is given at point X on the vertical axis as 17 mmHg. Linnér (1958) provides the increase in episcleral venous pressure as 1.25 mmHg. The facility of outflow can now be calculated from Equation 3.55:

$$C = \frac{(2.375 \ \mu l/min)}{[(30.5 - 17 - 1.25) \ mmHg]}$$

$$= \left(\frac{0.194 \ \mu l}{min \ mmHg}\right)$$

If no changes occur in aqueous humor production, outflow resistance, or episcleral venous pressure, the facility of outflow will be the same at all values of IOP. Unfortunately, an increase in IOP can decrease aqueous humor production, possibly by reducing the flow of that portion of aqueous, if any, due simply to filtration. *Pseudofacility* (Bill and Barany 1966) is the term used to describe the excess portion of "facility of outflow" in the measurement of C due to a *decrease* in aqueous humor *production* secondary to an increase in IOP.

Prijot (1961) studied the facility for human eyes using a tonographic method. His data (Figure 3.36) show that human facility is distributed about a mean of 0.25 μl/min mmHg. Other data suggest that the facility is 0.25 to 0.30 μl/min mmHg for the rabbit.

Since facility is a measure of the resistance to aqueous outflow from the eye, it is appropriate to inquire as to the site of this resistance. The most obvious location would be expected to be the trabecular meshwork and the inner wall of Schlemm's canal. Some recent studies, however, indicate that most of the resistance to flow is in the episcleral veins, but contradictory evidence exists. If the main resistance is in the episcleral veins, then the depth of the anterior chamber should have no effect on IOP, short of mechanically closing the angle entirely. Eyes with shallow anterior chambers, however, are clinically known to have lower values for facility, and deeper chambers, in myopes for example, are associated with higher facility values.

Effects of certain drugs also shed some light on the source of outflow resistance. Drugs that tend to dissolve out a portion of the trabecular meshwork increase facility; for example, Barany (1959) has shown that hyaluronidase, an enzyme that removes the gel-like hyaluronic acid from the meshwork, increases facility. This increase in facility is greater in eyes with wide angles than in eyes with shallow angles, suggesting that there is some additional resistance to aqueous

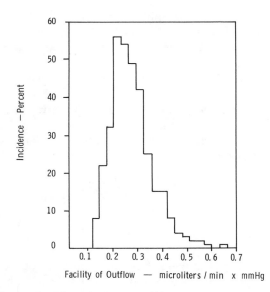

Figure 3.36 Incidence of outflow facility values in the human population. (From Davson H [ed.] [1969]: The Eye, Vol. 1. New York, Academic Press.)

outflow in the eyes with shallower angles. Pilocarpine, a drug commonly used to lower IOP, contracts the ciliary muscle and presumably opens the trabecular meshwork by mechanical stretching.

OTHER FACTORS INFLUENCING INTRAOCULAR PRESSURE

As already described, IOP is controlled by the rate of aqueous humor production and the resistance to its outflow. The production mechanism may be disturbed in many ways.

Production of aqueous humor occurs across the so-called blood–aqueous barrier. This term refers to that tissue in the ciliary epithelium separating blood plasma from aqueous humor; recall from the discussion in Chapter 2 that aqueous humor is not a simple blood filtrate. If this barrier is broken by any of several mechanisms, then protein, which is normally excluded from the aqueous humor, appears in the anterior chamber and is clinically seen as "flare." Flare is the simple scattering of light by the protein colloids that have now leaked into the aqueous humor. Certain chemical agents (nitrogen mustard and organic phosphates are examples) will damage epithelial cells and break down the blood–aqueous barrier to produce flare.

Mechanical injury or physical puncture of the eye may also lead to flare. Dilation of the blood vessels of the anterior uvea follows such trauma, and these capillaries may then exude a protein-rich solution into the anterior chamber. The rapid fall in IOP when fluid is lost from a penetrating wound (paracentesis) may create a stretching of the blood–aqueous barrier so that secretion and possible ultrafiltration mechanisms are overwhelmed by simple inflow of plasma.

For example, if a rabbit eye is emptied of aqueous humor, it will be refilled with fluid in about 30 minutes. This rate is much too fast to be attributed to secretion alone because the normal production rate is only about 1 to 3 µl/min; at that rate the replacement of 200 to 250 µl of aqueous humor would take about 2 hours.

Several osmotic pressure effects can be demonstrated in the eye, and some of these are clinically useful as well. The aqueous humor, for example, has a higher concentration of dissolved substances than does blood filtrate, so it would be expected that the eye would act as an osmometer (see Figure 2.3) (1) if the eye fluids were a stagnant system and (2) if the blood–aqueous barrier were a perfect semipermeable membrane. The aqueous humor is about 5 mOsm more concentrated than blood plasma; this concentration difference would lead to an osmotic IOP of 94 mmHg by Equation 2.1. The actual intraocular osmotic pressure, however, is much lower. Because the blood–aqueous barrier is not a perfect semipermeable membrane in a stagnant system, the leakage of solute across the imperfect semipermeable membrane will eventually equalize the concentrations inside and outside the barrier, and the pressure difference will fall toward zero. Some work must therefore be done in the eye to replenish lost solute; this is the active transport mechanism of the ciliary epithelium. The solute is transferred, or secreted, across the blood–aqueous barrier as a concentrated solution. There is then an osmotic flow of water that follows from the concentration gradient established across the barrier. The effect of the drug Diamox (acetazolamide) in reducing IOP is most likely obtained by its ability to inhibit this active transport mechanism.

This osmotic flow rate may be manipulated for clinical purposes. In acute angle-closure glaucoma, when the entrance to Schlemm's canal is blocked, it is essential to lower IOP quickly to avoid ocular damage. This can be done by raising the osmolarity of the blood plasma with a solute that does not cross, or only slowly crosses, the blood–aqueous barrier (and is only slowly removed by the kidneys so as to maintain its activity long enough to be effective). Urea, glycerol, and mannitol in large doses have all been used for this purpose. These materials, when they appear in the ocular blood vessels, cause an osmotic flow of fluid from the eye to the blood. Both aqueous and vitreous humor appear to be extracted, causing a large decrease in ocular volume and a subsequent drop in IOP. It must be emphasized that it is not necessary to have a perfect semipermeable membrane between the blood and the ocular fluids; an imperfect membrane will serve, although the effect may be smaller than if a perfect semipermeable membrane were present.

The movement of water into the eye from abnormally diluted blood plasma is used in the so-called water-provocative test for glaucoma. A patient suspected of having glaucoma drinks 1 liter of water quickly, after fasting. This makes the blood plasma temporarily more dilute than the aqueous humor, and the osmotic flow of water into the eye is increased. If the outflow channels for aqueous humor are open, the extra amount of aqueous humor quickly drains out, and there is little or no increase in IOP. If, however, the outflow channels are partially blocked, IOP rises (an increase of 8 mmHg is suggestive of glaucoma), falling only slowly as the excess aqueous drains through the abnormally resistant outflow channels.

4

The Vitreous Body

The vitreous body is a clear gel-like structure that fills the major portion of the internal volume of the eye. In humans, 60% of the globe is filled by the vitreous body, but in the rabbit, because of a relatively larger lens, only 30% of the volume of the eye is occupied by the vitreous. The vitreous body is the largest homogenous piece of intercellular material available from the mammalian body.

The gel-like vitreous body is currently considered to be a connective tissue with a very high water content (about 99%) and almost no cellular elements. It is directly in the optical path between the lens and the retina (see Figure 1.1). The vitreous body must be maintained in a relatively clear state for functional reasons. Its gel properties may aid in the maintenance of optical clarity by reducing the development of floating debris, as would likely appear if the vitreous were completely a liquid. The vitreous does become more liquid during the aging progress, and condensations (floaters) appear from a variety of processes, some normal and some pathological.

On one hand, the high water content of the vitreous body keeps it from being a barrier, greater than that of an equal volume of water, to the diffusive and convective movement of small molecules required for the nutrition of the surrounding tissues. The loose internal gel structure of the vitreous body, on the other hand, offers much more resistance to bulk water flow than would be present in a free body of water, but not so much as to prevent all circulation and movement of fluids in the vitreous chamber.

ANATOMY OF THE VITREOUS BODY

The vitreous body occupies the internal volume of the eye from the posterior surface of the lens to the anterior surface of the retina. There appears to be a membrane surrounding the entire outer surface of the vitreous body. This membrane is not comparable to a cell membrane in structure but is instead simply a region where the internal fibers of the vitreous body are more densely packed. An important portion of this membrane is that area covering the anterior portion of the vitreous body; this is known as the *anterior hyaloid membrane.*

The posterior surface of the vitreous body is in contact with the internal limiting membrane of the retina. The retina and the vitreous body can be easily separated when the globe is opened at its equator. There is evidence, however, that fibers from the vitreous body enter the retina to form a loose attachment. This attachment is somewhat stronger about the optic disk and very strong in an area (about 1.5 mm wide) immediately adjacent to the ora serrata known as the *vitreous base;* the vitreous cannot be peeled away or separated from the retina at this area.

One might expect little or no internal structure in a tissue composed of 99% water and 1% solids. Biomicroscopic examination, however, shows a tube-like (or tunnel-shaped) structure, known as the *canal of Cloquet,* running straight back from the center of the posterior lens to the optic disk. Although previously believed to be only an optical effect, it now seems clear that the canal of Cloquet is a zone formed by the internal fibrillar structure of the vitreous. This canal represents the remains of a blood vessel that ran from the optic nerve head to the lens in the embryo but that usually disappears by birth.

The cells of the vitreous appear to be concentrated in a thin layer, not more than 100 μm thick, at its outer surface. Cells are most numerous over the anterior surface of the vitreous, particularly at its base near the ciliary body and pars plana. Balazs and co-workers (1964) named these cells *hyalocytes.* The function of these cells is not clear, although they seem metabolically active; it has been suggested that they produce the hyaluronic acid (a glycosaminoglycan) of the vitreous body or are phagocytes (scavengers) of any foreign material that may appear in the vitreous.

CHEMICAL PROPERTIES OF THE VITREOUS BODY

The vitreous body is composed of three major structural components: water, collagen-like fibers, and glycosaminoglycans (GAGs). Ninety-nine percent of the weight of the vitreous body is water, and all the solids combined form the remaining 1% of weight. The most important solid moieties are proteins, which provide 0.08% of the vitreous mass (one-third as fibers and the remainder soluble), and the GAGs, which provide 0.02% to 0.05% of the mass and form the gel. GAGs are negatively charged sugar-like polymers; chemical structures of two ocular GAGs are shown in Figure 4.1. The remainder of the solid content of the vitreous consists largely of the salts normally found in body fluids.

When the vitreous body is dissected from the globe and placed on a filter paper, a clear colorless fluid drips out; this is the *vitreous humor* or *vitreous filtrate.* Remaining behind on the filter paper is a mass composed of the collapsed insoluble fibrous protein network. Some of the GAGs must also remain behind as there is evidence that the fibers are coated with this material. The vitreous humor is very similar to the aqueous humor in chemical composition; this observation supports the hypothesis (discussed below) that there is a movement of fluid from the anterior and posterior chambers into the vitreous body.

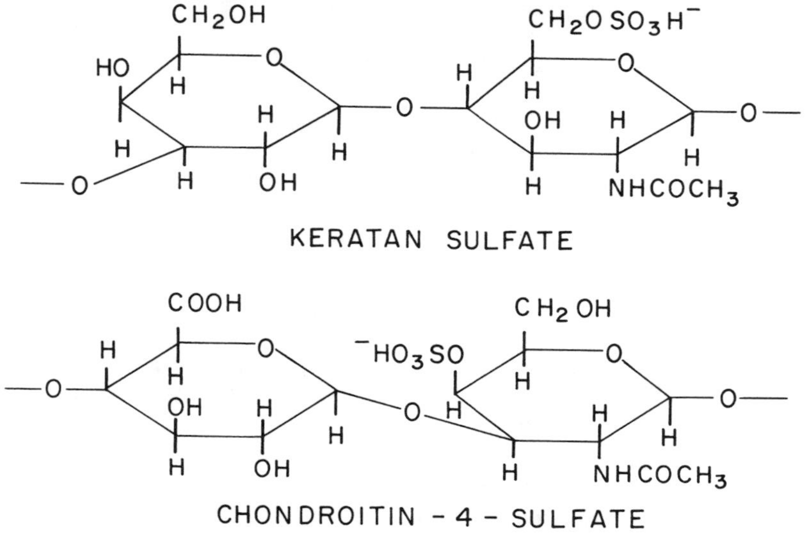

Figure 4.1 Chemical structure of two mucopolysaccharides found in the eye. Molecular weight is in the range 100,000 to 1,000,000; length ranges from 150 nm to 200 nm; diameter ranges from 1 nm to 10 nm.

The fibrous proteins of the vitreous body are probably collagen. There seems to be an interesting difference in that the vitreous body fibers in most mammals have bands spaced about 20 nm apart, whereas true collagen has bands spaced 64 nm apart. One report, however, suggests that the vitreous fibers in the cow are banded at this more normal 64-nm separation.

The fibers of the vitreous body are not cross-linked to form a solid three-dimensional structure. The fibers form a loose mesh in which each fiber is coated with GAGs. These GAG-covered fibers form a water-binding network. The importance of GAGs to the water content of the vitreous is easily demonstrated by noting the effects of cationic dyes or quaternary ammonium salts (e.g., cetylpyridinium chloride), which precipitate GAGs. There is a complete collapse of the vitreous body when such a chemical is applied, because the water quickly drains away.

The relative amounts of collagen fibers and GAGs have an important effect on the observed properties of the vitreous body. The vitreous body is very solid in frog and hen eyes, for example, where there are high collagen and low GAG contents. Conversely, in some primate eyes (e.g., the bush baby and owl monkey) there is little collagen but a large amount of GAG, leading to a more liquid vitreous. It appears that, although GAG can trap water, the system cannot become rigid unless the GAG–water complex is itself held in a collagen fiber meshwork. The interfibrillary spacing has been estimated to be about 2 μm (2000 nm). The total system is sufficiently close-knit so that, unlike a simple liquid, it can resist a shearing force.

The soluble protein content of the vitreous body is normally very small and does not scatter light. During paracentesis or inflammation, however, the soluble protein content may increase sufficiently to cause turbidity, similar to the observation of aqueous flare in the anterior chamber during such events.

The oxygen tension of the vitreous has been measured at about 20 mmHg polarographically by a number of authors in several mammals, and this tension increases closer to the retina.

PHYSICAL PROPERTIES
Osmosis

The response of the vitreous body to changes in osmotic pressure of the surrounding fluids is still unclear. Duke-Elder (1930) has shown that the vitreous body will absorb water as a function of the water vapor pressure of its surroundings. This water absorption is partially a swelling phenomenon, related to the presence of the GAG (we will see this activity again later in the corneal stroma), and partially an osmotic phenomenon caused by dissolved solids in the vitreous humor.

Although some investigators have proposed that the vitreous is surrounded by a semipermeable membrane, the evidence for this hypothesis is unconvincing. Kapetansky and Higbee (1969) have shown that the isolated vitreous body shrinks when placed for 15 minutes in a solution of 50% glycerol, whereas it swells in distilled water. The glyerol solution has a water-vapor pressure equivalent to a relative humidity of about 80%, but Duke-Elder (1930) showed that the water in equilibrium with the vitreous body at this humidity will be only 1/300 of that present in a fully saturated (100% relative humidity) water-vapor atmosphere. Kapetansky and Higbee should, therefore, have noted almost complete dehydration of the vitreous body instead of the 38% weight loss observed. They may not have allowed for full equilibrium (i.e., 15 minutes is a short time period) or glycerol may have penetrated into the vitreous body under study. When the vitreous body was moved from the glycerol to distilled water, the weight regain was about 11% in an additional 15 minutes. This is not surprising as it is simply a reversal of the dehydration process carried out in the glycerol solution. Neither the glycerol nor the distilled water tests give any evidence for a semipermeable membrane around the vitreous body.

In vivo studies by Robbins and Galen (1969) have shown that orally administered glycerol and intravenously administered urea and mannitol cause reductions in vitreous body weight in the rabbit. This is not surprising as the vitreous is in close contact with the internal vascular beds of the eye and any changes in osmotic pressure in the vessels will cause a transient osmotic flow of water. Again, it is not necessary to postulate a true semipermeable barrier around the vitreous body. The presence of such a barrier can only be proved by observing water flow under a steady-state osmotic imbalance; an osmotic imbalance in the transient state can induce the flow of water even in the absence of a semipermeable membrane.

Flow Conductivity

Flow conductivity is the term used in the ophthalmic literature to describe the ability of water molecules to move as a liquid phase. An important distinction should be made between convection in a liquid and convective flow in a gel. Convection in a liquid refers to the swirling movement of the liquid in response to thermal gradients or mechanical stirring. Convective (or "bulk") flow in a gel is a slow movement of fluid down a pressure gradient.

As the vitreous body is a connective tissue of 99% water content, it would be expected to allow passage of water under a hydrostatic pressure gradient. The movement of the vitreous humor through the vitreous body, however, poses an interesting but as yet incompletely resolved problem. Hayreh (1966) made a thorough review of past work and added his own observations. He concluded, from studies using colloidal iron as a tracer of movement, that there was considerable flow of liquid posterior through the rabbit vitreous body.

The measurements of Brubaker and Riley (1972) on excised samples of rabbit vitreous body can be used to estimate the ability of water to move through this tissue when a hydrostatic pressure gradient is applied. First, flow conductivity is the proportionality constant in *Darcy's law* that relates the flow rate to the applied hydrostatic pressure gradient. For a membrane

$$\frac{dv}{dt} = K \, a \left(\frac{\Delta P}{L} \right) \tag{4.1}$$

where dv/dt is the flow rate in volume/time, a is the surface area of the membrane, ΔP is the pressure drop across the membrane, and L is the membrane thickness. K is the flow conductivity term, which includes the viscosity of the flowing fluid; that is

$$K = \frac{k}{u} \tag{4.2}$$

where k is the contribution of the internal pore geometry and u is the fluid viscosity. This will be discussed in greater detail in Chapter 6.

Brubaker and Riley (1972) gave the flow conductivity (K) of the rabbit vitreous body as 1.5×10^{-9} cm^4 dyne^{-1} sec^{-1}. A later reinvestigation gave a slightly different value of 3 to 6×10^{-9} cm^4 dyne^{-1} sec^{-1} for rabbit and steer vitreous body (Fatt 1977a). The flow conductivity of human corneal stroma, for comparison, was found to be 17×10^{-13} cm^4 dyne^{-1} sec^{-1} (Fatt and Hedbys 1970a), scleral flow conductivity was found to be 15×10^{-13} cm^4 dyne^{-1} sec^{-1} (Fatt and Hedbys 1970b), and retina flow conductivity was measured at 9.4×10^{-9} cm^4 dyne^{-1} sec^{-1} (Fatt and Shantinath 1971).

Bert and Fatt (1970) have described a theoretical model of the structure of swelling connective tissue that allows the internal pore structure to be estimated from flow conductivity. Their model predicts that the water-filled spaces between the long-chain GAG molecules in the vitreous body will permit passage of particles up to 130 nm in diameter. This crude estimate is supported by studies of light scattering and double refraction during flow of GAG solutions, which indicate a molecule 1 to 10 nm in diameter and 200 nm long; it is not unreasonable to assume a gel composed of these molecules would have pores of 130-nm diameter. Such large pores would also explain the success various investigators have had using colloidal particles as tracers of water movement in the vitreous body.

If the vitreous body had a simple geometric shape, the convective flow could be calculated directly from the flow conductivity and applied pressure gradient using a rearrangement of Equation 4.1 (Darcy's law):

$$\frac{(dv/dt)}{a} = K \frac{dP}{dx} \tag{4.3}$$

where $(dv/dt)/a$ is the flow rate per unit area, K is the flow conductivity, and dP/dx is the gradient of hydraulic pressure. The simplest hypothesis is that intraocular pressure is applied at the anterior hyaloid membrane adjacent to the zonule and lens. The geometry of the internal eye, however, is too complex to allow an analytical solution of this problem.

An alternative method was therefore used by Fatt and Rosenbluth in an unpublished experiment. They employed a complex electrolytic copper-tank model to apply Darcy's law to the eye. A fairly good approximation to the geometry of the vitreous body is shown in Figure 4.2. The vitreous–retinal interface is approximated by the section of a sphere S, and the zonule–vitreous interface is approximated by a disk Z into which is set a segment of a sphere L, which represents the lens–vitreous interface. The model eye (Figure 4.3) was filled with an electrolyte solution (KCl), and a voltage drop was applied between areas L to Z and the shell S. The conductivity of the KCl solution can be measured and is analogous to the flow conductivity of the vitreous. Current, which was measured, is analogous to fluid flow, and the voltage drop is analogous to the pressure drop between the IOP (at the anterior surface of the vitreous body) and the pressure at the outer surface of the sclera. This is the method that was used to predict that aqueous outflow along the uveoscleral route was about 20% of the total, as discussed in Chapter 3. Fatt and Hedbys (1970b) previously estimated that 21% of the aqueous outflow in humans occurred through the sclera, and Kleinstein and Fatt (1977) experimentally found a trans-scleral flow of aqueous humor of 0.3 μl/min in the living rabbit; this is about 10% of the aqueous humor production rate of the rabbit as given by Maurice (1959).

It is also desirable to know how the flow is distributed in the vitreous body and over the surface of the sclera. Seven disk electrodes were inserted into the shell S of the model eye. Current could be measured at all these loci, and Figure 4.4 was drawn showing the resultant lines of isopotential (i.e., isopressure) and corresponding perpendicular lines of electrical (i.e., fluid) flow. Fatt and Rosenbluth also checked their electrolytic tank model against a complex mathematical analysis and found good agreement.

Finally, this same model was used to predict the diffusion of solutes in the vitreous. The results of Fatt (1975), which showed that solute transport in the vitreous is the sum of both diffusion and convective (bulk) flow, were used to

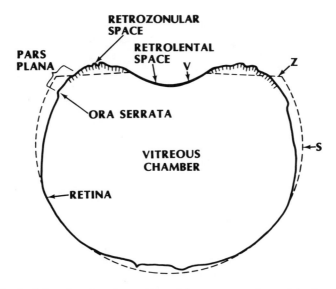

Figure 4.2 Dashed line showing the outline of the copper-tank model when it is superimposed on a cross-section of the human vitreous body.

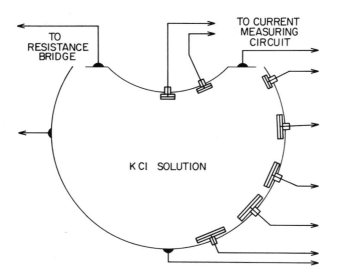

Figure 4.3 Cross-section of the copper tank that served as a model of the vitreous body of the human eye.

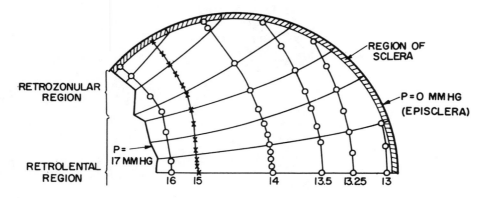

Figure 4.4 Isopotentials and stream flow lines in the vitreous body as they were obtained from the copper tank that served as a model of the human eye in Figure 4.3. The curves with circles and crosses are curves of constant pressure, starting with the imposed 17 mmHg in the retrolental space and decreasing to 13 mmHg at the retina. The pressure at the outer surface of the sclera was taken as 0 mmHg. The curves at right angles to the isopotentials are streamlines that show the path of intraocular fluid (aqueous humor) as it flows from the retrolental space toward the retina.

compare the carrying capacity of solutes by convective flow—directed toward the posterior under hydraulic pressure—to that of diffusion—directed from any area of high concentration to any area of low concentration. This comparison indicated that diffusion is by far the dominant force in the vitreous where the movement of small molecules is concerned. Therefore, the experimental observation of Maurice (1957a) that radioactive sodium ions injected into the vitreous body behind the lens eventually appear in the anterior chamber does not contradict the conclusion that there is a posteriorly directed liquid flow in the vitreous body driven by intraocular pressure. Fatt (1975) has indicated that small ions or molecules with large diffusion coefficients could diffuse anteriorly despite a very slow posterior-ward liquid flow in the vitreous body. Large particles, on the other hand, such as those used by Fowlks and associates (1963) and others, when deposited in the vitreous body would diffuse so slowly that they would be carried posteriorly.

Several of the authors mentioned above have suggested a potential role for the posterior movement of fluid and materials through the vitreous in the nutrition of the retina. The total needs of the retina may be satisfied by delivery of metabolites, including oxygen, via both the vitreous and the blood circulatory system.

5

The Lens

The crystalline lens and the cornea together form the compound lens that projects the optical image on the retina. Although the lens has more curvature and is thicker than the cornea, it has only one-half the refracting power of the cornea. The functionally low refractive power of the lens is a consequence of the very small change in refractive index at its surfaces *in vivo*. Within the eye, the lens is bathed by the aqueous humor at its anterior surface and is in contact with the vitreous body at the posterior surface; the refractive indices of the aqueous humor–lens–vitreous body are respectively 1.336:1.39:1.336 according to Emsley (1963). The cornea makes a greater contribution to the total refractive power of the eye as a consequence of both its curvature (approximately 7.8 mm) and high refractive index (1.376) compared to that of air (index of 1.0).

Although the lens provides only about 30% of the refracting power of the eye, it provides all of the focusing power. The lens remains in a fixed position within the eye (in mammals), but its thickness and surface curvatures vary to change the focus of light.

Properties of the lens of interest from the standpoint of vegetative physiology are (1) its elasticity, (2) its transparency, (3) its nutrition and growth as an avascular tissue, (4) its ion transport, and (5) changes in its composition with age and in states of disease.

STRUCTURE

The lens is a biconvex semisolid. It appears transparent in the human, with perhaps a slightly yellowish tinge that is just noticeable in the lens of the newborn but increases with age. The geometric centers of its convex surfaces are called the *anterior* and *posterior poles,* and the rounded junction of these two convex surfaces is called the *equator.* The anterior pole is about 3 mm behind the posterior corneal surface in humans. The human lens has a diameter of 9 to 10 mm and a thickness of 4 to 5 mm, both dimensions varying as the eye is focused for far or near objects. The anterior surface is a segment of a sphere about 9 mm in radius, whereas the posterior surface has a radius of curvature approximately 6 mm

(Hogan et al. 1971) These parameters vary in individuals and with age and state of accommodation. Irregular linear structures, called *sutures,* may be seen within the lens, radiating outward from the center. The sutures are believed to be the result of the growth of the long cells that form the lens.

The lens is composed of a mass of these elongated cells, called *lens fibers* (Figure 5.1), and is enclosed in the *lens capsule.* The capsule, an elastic collagen membrane containing some glycosamines, is produced as a basement membrane by the *lens epithelium,* a single layer of cuboidal cells just under the capsule at its anterior face. These epithelial cells are the origin for all the fibers. The mature fiber is in the shape of a long, thin ribbon with a flattened but roughly hexagonal cross-section. Each ribbon is 7 to 10 mm long, 8 to 10 μm wide, and 2 to 5 μm thick. The fibers fit together to form smooth lamellae in radial rows, parallel to the curved surfaces of the lens. The cells are interlocked with "tongue and groove" interdigitations along their long sides, which prevents the cells from sliding across one another (Hogan et al. 1971). The new cells near the anterior pole of the lens are cuboidal. As they are pushed toward the equator, however, the cells elongate and begin to take on the form of the lens fibers described earlier. Younger fibers are laid down on top of older ones, and the older fibers become more dense and tightly packed as the lens grows around them. The earliest fibers, at the center of the lens, form the *nucleus,* whereas the newer fibers laid down near the surface form the lens *cortex.* The result is a soft cortex with a hard nucleus. The sutures are formed on both polar surfaces where the fibers meet.

All the cells of the lens are derived from the epithelium, and so all parts of the lens are composed of the same kind of cells but of different age. No cells are

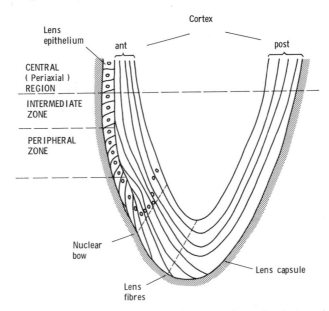

Figure 5.1 Schematic drawing of a meridional section through a human lens.

ever shed by the lens; therefore, all the cells laid down while the individual was an embryo and all cells formed thereafter are present in the adult lens. The human lens continues to grow throughout life, with the rate of formation of new cells being high in the newborn and young persons but decreasing with aging. The increase in size from newborn to adulthood maintains the density as a constant, but thereafter the lens density increases. The weight of the human lens consequently increases linearly with age (Figure 5.2).

The chemical composition of the lens is not the same in all portions. The average composition of the lens, however, is about 63% water; 36% protein; and 1% lipids, salts, and carbohydrates. For comparison, the blood plasma contains 6% protein, the inside of the red blood cell is about 40% protein, and the corneal stroma is about 20% protein. The protein content of the lens increases toward its center; cortex cells are 27% protein, whereas nuclear cells are 40% protein. Lens proteins have been broadly grouped into both insoluble (*"albuminoid"*; about 12% of the total protein) and soluble proteins; the latter are divided into alpha (molecular weight of 8×10^5; about 30% of total protein), beta (molecular weight of 28×10^3; about 50% of total protein), and gamma (molecular weight varying from 14 to 25×10^3; only about 1% of total protein) crystallins; further subdivisions have been proposed, but these are beyond the scope of this text.

Nuclei and organelles (mitochondria and microsomes) are relatively sparse in lens cells. For example, the nucleus and organelles of the calf lens cell account for only 4% of its total protein, whereas about 50% of the calf liver cell proteins are concentrated in its nucleus and organelles. Also, nucleated cells are found only in the most peripheral layers of the lens. The relatively small number of organelles in the lens cell contributes to lens transparency because the size of these organelles

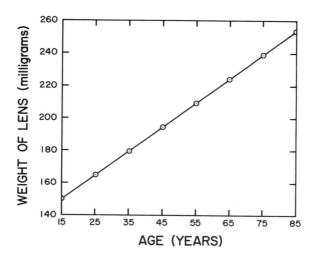

Figure 5.2 Weight of the human lens as a function of age.

(about 500 nm [0.5 μm]) would be sufficient to give appreciable scattering to light if organelles were present in large numbers, whereas proteins are smaller in size and produce less scattering (see later).

ACCOMMODATION AND ELASTICITY

The lens changes its shape during the process of focusing optical images on the retina. It is thicker when the eye is focused on near objects and thinner when focused on far objects. The change in thickness and curvature is accomplished by means of the suspensory ligament, called the *zonule of Zinn* (Figure 5.3). Scanning electron microscope study (Rohen 1979) indicates that the zonular fibers form an interconnected mat attached to the ciliary epithelium of the pars plana. This mat is organized into sagittally oriented plates running in the ciliary valleys and closely attached to the lateral walls of the ciliary processes. Where the zonular fibers leave the ciliary valleys and run toward the lens capsule, there is an abrupt change in their direction (Figure 5.4). At this bend a set of fine fibrils, called *span* or *tension fibers,* continue forward and attach firmly.

Helmholtz (in *Treatise on Physiological Optics*) described the theory of the mechanism of accommodation that is still accepted today. When the ciliary muscle, to which the other end of the zonular fibers are connected, is relaxed, the zonule is under tension and pulls on the equatorial edge of the lens capsule to give a thin lens, focused for distant objects. As the ciliary muscle contracts, the ciliary body moves forward and inward, bulging where the tension fibers are attached. These fibers take up the tension, allowing the zonule to relax. This process releases the tension on the equatorial region of the lens capsule, and the natural elasticity of this capsule causes the lens to round and thicken, focusing the eye for nearer objects.

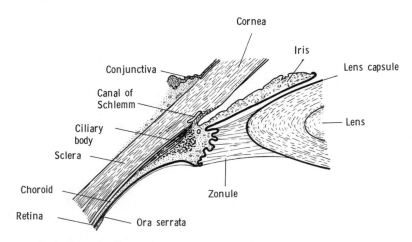

Figure 5.3 Anteroposterior section through the anterior portion of a human eye.

The elasticity is most likely in the lens capsule rather than in the interior portion of the lens. The high water content of the lens makes it almost incompressible. The cortex is a semiliquid gel and is therefore not able to withstand shear stresses. The hard nucleus deeply buried in the soft cortex is unlikely to contribute to the observed elasticity of the lens. By elimination, therefore, the elasticity must be a property of the capsule.

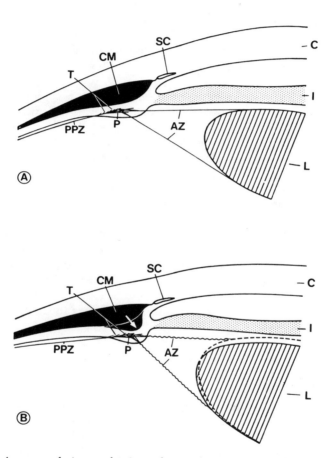

Figure 5.4 Accommodative mechanism schema. *A,* nonaccommodating eye: ciliary muscle (*CM*) relaxed; anterior zonular fibers (*AZ*) stretched by traction from posterior (pars plana) zonular fibers (*PPZ*); lens (*L*) flattened. B, accommodating eye: ciliary muscle contracted, forming an inner edge; the tension fiber system (*T*) is stretched, taking up the traction from posterior zonular fibers and the choroid. Thus, the anterior zonular fibers become relaxed, and the lens becomes more spherical (*dotted lines*). *P,* Zonular plexus; *I,* iris; *C,* cornea; *SC,* Schlemm's canal. Arrow indicates direction of ciliary muscle movement during accommodation. (From Rohen JW [1979]: Scanning electron microscopic studies of the zonular apparatus in human and monkey eyes. Invest. Ophthalmol. Vis. Sci. 18 (2):133–144. With permission.)

Because the lens is incompressible, its volume must remain the same no matter what shape it assumes. If the lens were a sphere of incompressible material, then its surface would be at a minimum for the volume it contains; if this sphere were flattened, the surface area would increase. Although the lens is not a true sphere, it can be shown geometrically that the two somewhat spherical segments that make up its surfaces must increase in radii of curvature as it is flattened, and therefore the capsule surface area must increase. A flattened lens therefore has a stretched capsule, and in this stretched membrane resides the elasticity of the lens. As tension in the zonule is relieved by contraction of the ciliary muscle, the capsule contracts and tends to give a lens of smaller surface area: that is, a thick lens with anterior and posterior surfaces of more spherical topography and shorter radii of curvature.

Humans begin to note an apparant decline in their accommodative ability after the age of 40 years, this difficulty is termed *presbyopia*. Koretz and Handelman (1988) offered a theory for presbyopia. They found that the older the individual, the more curved the lens becomes for a given accommodative demand; this is necessary because the refractive index of the lens decreases with aging, perhaps related to the known shift in its protein from soluble to insoluble form (Spector 1984). The increase in curvature compensates for decreased refractive index. Additional internal compensatory changes in refraction may also exist (related to the clinically observed "zones of discontinuity" that are seen within the lens). From mathematical modeling, Koretz and Handelman also found that the angle of zonular insertion should change with increasing lenticular size, weakening its effectiveness. As the lens increases in size with aging, the zonules come to exert a force that is tangential (or nearly so) to the surface of the lens so that zonular relaxation has less and less effect on the shape of the lens. Eventually, the compensatory mechanisms described above begin to fail, and then the lens system slowly loses its accommodative abilities.

TRANSPARENCY

The transparency of the lens must simply be a consequence of the low number of scattering centers (perhaps the organelles). The lens cell is composed largely of protein molecules, about 10 nm in diameter, in colloidal solution. The particle size is sufficiently small and the concentration is sufficiently low that scattering, although present, reduces the transmission of white light only a few percentage units (Figure 5.5) (Bettelheim and Ali 1985). The increase in scattering with age may be a result of aggregation of the proteins into insoluble, larger particles.

The layers of the lens have different refractive indices. This change is not gradual; there is a stepwise increase toward the interior (Davson 1969). The refractive index is close to 1.38 in the cortex, but rises to 1.40 in the nucleus as a consequence of the increasing protein content mentioned earlier.

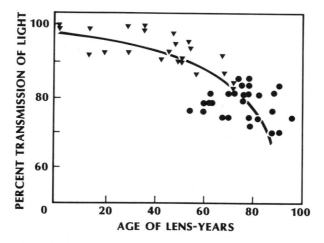

Figure 5.5 Age dependence of percent transmission of white unpolarized light. ▼ Normal lenses; ● cataractous lenses. Curve represents a polynomial fitted to all data points. (From Bettelheim FA, Chylack LT [1985]: Light scattering of whole excised human cataractous lenses. Relationships between different light scattering parameters. Exp. Eye Res. 41:19–30. With permission.)

METABOLISM AND NUTRITION

The lens becomes a completely avascular tissue shortly after its very early embryonic state. All nutrients and oxygen for cell respiration must come from the aqueous humor or through the vitreous body. Conversely, all waste products must be transported or diffuse out of the lens in order to be carried away by the aqueous humor or through the vitreous.

The energy released by the metabolic processes of the lens (the reaction of oxygen with glucose) is used in several ways. Energy is used to synthesize large, high-energy molecules (proteins), to maintain the temperature of the tissue, and to continue the active transportation of ions or uncharged molecules against osmotic or electrochemical gradients.

The lens is continuously making new cells and needs protein for this process. Merriam and Kinsey (1950) showed that radioactive amino acids were combined to form lens proteins when whole calf lens was incubated *in vitro* with tissue-culture techniques. Protein synthesis was not uniform over the entire lens but seemed to be at a high rate at the equatorial and anterior regions and at a low rate, if at all, in the posterior area and nucleus. Research on ox lens also indicates less protein synthesis in the nucleus than in the cortex. *In vivo* studies on rat lens have shown, moreover, that a single injected dose of radioactive amino acid is incorporated into the protein of the outer fiber layer of cells, particularly those at the lens equator. As time progresses, these labelled fibers are found to be deeper within the lens.

Energy production depends on the supply of both glucose and oxygen. Measurements have shown that essentially all the oxygen uptake of the lens is by the cells of the cortex. Oxygen consumption of the cortex alone is 0.15 μl/mg dry weight per hour, whereas the entire lens has been shown to consume 0.10 μl/mg dry weight per hour. As the nucleus is known to have almost zero consumption of oxygen, these two measurements indicate that the cortex contains about two-thirds of the total dry solids of the lens.

Glucose consumption has been found to be 3 to 5 mg/day in rabbit lens. About 80% of this glucose is converted to lactic acid in the lens. This means that lens cells are acting as though they were not receiving sufficient oxygen for complete aerobic metabolism. This may be a consequence of inadequate oxygen supply through the aqueous humor, since delivery is limited by diffusion. On the other hand, the oxygen tension in the aqueous is most likely about 50 to 70 mmHg, and this is felt to be the equivalent of tissue oxygen tension found elsewhere. The presence of anaerobic metabolism in the lens, therefore, and in the cornea as well (see Chapter 7), remains unexplained.

Lens cells may also make a very small amount of glycogen by removing water from glucose via the reaction

$$C_6H_{12}O_6 - H_2O => C_6H_{10}O_5$$

Glycogen can be stored as an emergency source of energy. Another means for the utilization of glucose by the lens is through the sorbitol pathway, in which glucose is converted to sorbitol by the enzyme aldose reductase. Sorbitol is then further converted to fructose by the enzyme polyol dehydrogenase. Although the functional significance of the sorbitol pathway has been the subject of much debate, it is still unclear (van Heyningen 1962; Kuck 1961).

Lens cells also synthesize lipids, as indicated by the relatively high lipid content of the lens: 2.5% of the wet weight, or 7.5% of the dry weight, of the lens is lipids.

Some of the metabolic energy produced by the lens cells from the oxidation of glucose is used to maintain an intracellular concentration of ions that is different from that found in the extracellular fluid. This is an almost universal phenomenon found in living cells, and examples are seen in nerves, muscles, and red blood cells and in the ciliary epithelium as described in Chapter 2. The reason for this energy expenditure in the instance of the lens is to maintain an osmotic balance favoring transparency. Metabolic poisons that interrupt this process cause osmotic swelling.

The lens fibers are lower in Na^+ and higher in K^+ concentration than is either the aqueous or vitreous humor. This separation, for which energy must be expended, is made across the lens cell membranes themselves rather than across the capsule; the isolated washed capsule is freely permeable to all molecules except those of very large size. Also, if the capsule is dissolved away by collagenase, the ion concentration power of the cells is unaffected. If the cells are cooled below 37°C or starved of glucose, however, then the concentration of Na^+ or K^+ approaches that of the aqueous humor. The effect of oxygen on ion concentrations depends on the presence of glucose. The withholding of oxygen from the lens in the absence of glucose will cause development of abnormal Na^+ and K^+ concentrations, but the lens cells can maintain their ion transport system by anaerobic metabolism in the presence of glucose.

Chemical analysis of the lens shows ion concentrations that are largely representative of the intracellular material because only 5% to 10% of the water in the lens is extracellular (or *between* the fibers). Table 5.1 shows the Na^+ and K^+ concentrations in both the lens and aqueous humor.

The high ion concentrations in the nucleus are a consequence of the low water content in this part of the lens. More informative than the simple concentrations is the Na^+-to-K^+ ratio, also shown in Table 5.1 (last column). The cortex is clearly more active than the nucleus in maintaining ion concentrations that are different from those of the bathing fluid. More detailed studies have supported the view that the epithelial cells are the most active portion of the lens cortex in transporting ions.

CATARACT

Aging in humans and other species is commonly accompanied by changes in the lens system leading to reduced accommodation (discussed earlier) and often a later loss in transparency. Any alteration of optical homogeneity or loss of transparency in the lens, especially if it reduces visual acuity, is termed a *cataract*. Cataracts of the lens may result from various causes other than solely aging, although this is the most common form.

Systemic metabolic diseases can induce cataracts. Diabetes, for example, often results in lenticular opacification through a complex and yet incompletely understood cascade of changes. Some individuals are born without the ability to produce an enzyme (galactose 1 phosphate-uridyl transferase) that metabolizes galactose, which is formed in the gastrointestinal tract by the breakdown of the lactose present in dairy products. After an individual consumes milk or other dairy foods, galactose increases in the circulatory system and finally appears in the aqueous humor. The increased galactose is converted to dulcitol by aldose reductase within the lens. Dulcitol, however, may not be further acted on by polyol dehydrogenase, so that it rapidly accumulates within the lens and then osmotically draws in water from the aqueous, resulting in a "galactose" cataract. If galactosemia is recognized promptly and dietary galactose is eliminated, the lens vacuoles may disappear.

Table 5.1 Concentrations of Na+ and K+ in the Lens and Aqueous Humor (mm/Liter)

	Na^+	K^+	Sum	K^+:Na^+
Ox cortex	54.5	90.1	144.6	1.650
Ox nucleus	90.0	120.6	210.6	1.350
Aqueous humor	147.0	4.9	151.9	0.033

Cataracts may be associated with other systemic diseases, such as congenital hemolytic anemia or homocystinuria; with the use of drugs (such as ophthalmic steroids) or other toxic substances (see Davson 1969 for a detailed discussion); with dietary deficiencies; and with hereditary errors of metabolism or development. Radiation is an important modern problem because such exposure may occur from accidental or therapeutic exposure of the head to x-rays, gamma rays or neutron beams. There is uncertainty about the effects of lower-energy electromagnetic radiation used in communications, radar, microwave appliances, and industrial devices. Infrared radiation has long been known to lead to "glassblowers' cataract," but the development of such changes is a slow process, requiring regular exposure over many years.

Spector (1984) suggests age-related or senescent (senile) cataracts occur because long-term oxidative insult subtly damages lens cell membranes, leading to ineffective transport functions. This in turn sets off changes in ion concentrations and increased adenosine triphosphate (ATP) utilization by competing ion transport systems within the lens. Less energy is available for non-pump metabolism such as protein synthesis. ATP levels fall, but glucose metabolism may be initially stimulated via glycolysis and the hexose monophosphate shunt. Oxidation in membrane polypeptides, glutathione, and cytosol proteins close to the cell membranes allow unfolding of these proteins, exposing additional groups susceptible to oxidation. Changes that occur include formulation of disulfide-linked aggregates, loss of metabolic activity, increased proteolysis, and a drop in ATP and possibly nicotinamide-adenine dinucleotide phosphate (NADPH) concentrations. Membrane permeability increases, causing loss of amino acids and other metabolites and general changes in ion content. Large protein aggregates develop, cell membranes rupture, low molecular weight protein and water content increases, and finally scattering increases (see Figure 5.5) and opacification occurs (Bettelheim and Chylack 1985). Some recent studies implicate exposure to ultraviolet radiation as a major contributing factor to the formation of age-related cataract (McDonagh and Nguyen 1989).

Cataracts are often divided into groups based on the location of the opacification: *nuclear* if the lesion is central, and *cortical* if the lesion is more peripheral. *Posterior subcapular cataracts* may disturb vision more than their clinical appearance would suggest. The age of onset, the degree of "maturity," the color (e.g., *brunescent* is used to describe a brown and usually senescent cataract), the etiology, and the degree and location of the opacification are also used to identify lenticular changes. Congenital cataracts can be *zonular;* these opacifications seem to occupy a zone or spherical lamella within the lens. Other congenital cataracts may be genetically determined or *secondary* to incomplete development (e.g., persistent hyperplastic primary vitreous) or disease (e.g., rubella). *Senescent* (senile) cataracts often begin with vacuoles or small opacities in the lens cortex or with changes in color or opacities in the nucleus. Water clefts and lamellar separations occur and can be termed *cuneiform* or *coronary* if these descriptive terms apply. The *morgagnian* cataract is one in which the cortex is milky and has liquefied so that the hard brown nucleus has sunk into an inferior position. *Hypermature* cataracts occur when the capsule begins to leak the liquefied cortex; the lens shrinks in volume, the surface wrinkles, and the debris that has now moved into the aqueous humor may secondarily stimulate inflammation and/or directly block the aqueous outflow, leading to glaucoma.

6

Cornea I: Form, Swelling Pressure, Transport Processes, and Optics*

The cornea and sclera together form the outer tunic of the eye and give the eye its shape. The cornea is the transparent section of this tunic and occupies about 7% of the total area of the globe in humans. The corneal portion is greater in lower animals: 25% in the rabbit and 50% in the rat.

The cornea is covered *in vivo* by a continually renewed watery film, the tears, to protect this highly specialized tissue from drying and from irritating contaminants in the air. The tear film also provides an excellent smooth optical surface to interface with the air (Chapter 10 discusses the tears in greater detail).

The combination of cornea and crystalline lens provides most of the light-focusing power of the eye. The cornea is the dominant partner in this collaboration, even though it is quite thin compared to the lens. The anterior surface of the cornea, covered by the tears, faces the air to give a refractive index change from the air to the cornea of 1.000 to 1.376. Roughly 70% of the total optical power of the eye is provided by this interface. The lens, although relatively thick and of steep curvature and high refractive index, is surrounded by fluid of almost equal refractive index and thus has reduced refractive effect.

Many properties of the cornea are of special interest because they relate in one way or another to the maintenance of corneal transparency. Among these are (1) tissue mechanical properties, (2) optical properties, (3) mass transfer properties, (4) nutrition, (5) response to changes in environment, and (6) growth and repair. Clinicians are interested in the corneal response to disease, laceration, abrasion, and blunt impact, and particularly to contact lens wear.

*Figures 6.2 to 6.6 are courtesy of Dr. Jan P. G. Bergmanson.

STRUCTURE

If the anterior portion of an imaginary perfectly spherical human eye (radius about 12 mm) were flattened or pulled inward, the cornea would be located on this portion. The mean central radius of curvature of the human cornea is shorter than the radius of the whole globe, averaging 7.86 mm (SD 0.26 mm), and about 1.5% larger in men than in women. This corneal radius of curvature is shorter in infants and neonates, whereas with keratoconus* a central portion of the cornea has become steep in radius, thin, and distorted. Normal corneal surface topography is more closely that of an ellipse than a sphere when the entire surface is considered. Additionally, many corneas are toric, having different curvatures in two major meridians 90° apart, producing refractive astigmatism.

In external examination of the human eye the outer surface of the cornea appears elliptical because of the inferior and superior anterior extensions of the opaque sclera. The major axis is horizontal and is about 11 to 12 mm long in 95% of eyes. When viewed from inside the eye, however, the cornea is a section of an almost perfect sphere with a diameter of about 11.7 mm. The external vertical minor axis is about 10.6 mm in length. External corneal axis lengths are about 1% longer in men than in women.

Corneal thickness in humans, measured *in vivo* with an optical pachometer attached to a slitlamp biomicroscope, is about 0.52 mm (SD 0.04 mm) in the central region, thickening in the periphery to about 0.65 mm. The thickness of the cornea is dependent on many factors, including osmolarity of the tears, oxygen supply, temperature, drug treatment, contact lens wear, and age. Because experimental animals play such a large part in corneal research, it is worth noting that the cornea in the ox is about 0.8 mm thick, in the cat about 0.6 mm thick, in the rabbit about 0.4 mm thick, and in the mouse about 0.1 mm thick (Maurice 1984).

The human cornea may be subdivided into five layers, excluding the covering tear film. The outermost of these is the *epithelium* (ectodermal in origin). *Bowman's membrane* is beneath, followed by the *stroma,* and finally *Descemet's membrane* and the *endothelium.* It is currently believed that much of the posterior cornea is derived from neural crest cells during fetal development.

The epithelium is a layer 5 to 7 cells deep and about 50 to 60 μm thick in humans (Figures 6.1 and 6.2). The epithelium is formed of more cellular layers near the limbus. One-third of this thickness (in the central cornea) is provided by a single sheet of *columnar* cells (about 20 μm high and 10 μm wide), forming the basal layer. These basal cells contact their neighbors along their lateral and anterior walls with numerous desmosomal junctions, whereas clusters of hemidesmosomes firmly anchor these cells to their underlying 40 to 50-nm thick *basement membrane.* Mitotic activity occurs in the basal layer. *Wing* (or "umbrella") cells, two or three layers deep, are derived from and cover the basal cells, and they flatten as they are pushed toward the corneal surface where there are two to three

---

*Keratoconus is a pathological condition of the eye in which the cornea becomes conical over a portion of its surface.

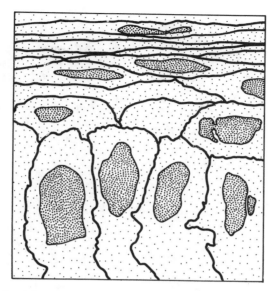

Figure 6.1 Sketch of the cross-sectional cellular structure of a normal rabbit epithelium based on an electron micrograph. The tissue is about 50 μm thick.

layers of stratified *squamous* cells. Shedding of these cells into the tear layer is their ultimate fate.

The large spherical nuclei of the basal cells flatten along with the entire cellular structure as the cells age, but unlike the stratified epithelial cells of the skin the squamous corneal cells do not normally become keratinized. The type and distribution of organelles (Golgi apparatus, endoplasmic reticulum, but only a few mitochondria) seen in the basal layer suggest low aerobic oxidation (Dohlman 1971), and these disappear as the epithelial cells evolve in form and location over a time period of about 1 week. Another feature of these surface cells is the large numbers of microplicae (up to 1 μm in length) and microvilli (0.5 μm tall, 0.3 μm wide, and 0.5 μm apart) covering their tear-side surface; these features may serve to anchor the tear layer to the corneal surface. The squamous cells are wide and thin, measuring 20 to 45 μm in width by 4 μm in thickness.

Lymphocytes and occasional macrophages may be found among the basal and wing cells, and dendritic polymorphous cells believed to be Langerhans cells have also been observed deep in the epithelial layer (Hogan et al. 1971; Bergmanson 1990).

Most corneal glucose consumption (perhaps 90%) occurs in the epithelium. Both the tricarboxylic acid (TCA) cycle and hexose-monophosphate shunt have been identified (Kinoshita et al. 1955). Stored glycogen is also found in the epithelium, and is known to be about 7% of the dry weight of the tissue in several species. Epithelial glycogen stores have been shown to decrease with contact lens wear. Contact lens wear also leads to a redistribution of epithelial

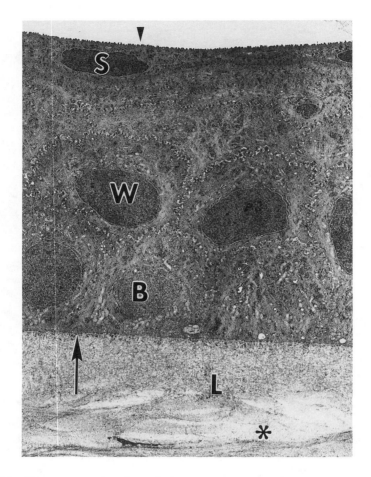

Figure 6.2 Transverse section through the anterior cornea. The compact, stratified corneal epithelium consists of basal (*B*), wing (*W*), and squamous (*S*) cells. Along its surface, microvilli (*triangle*) are projecting into the tears. Internally the epithelium is adherent to its basement membrane (*arrow*), which posteriorly faces the collagenous anterior limiting lamina (*L*). The stroma (or substantia propria) (*asterisk*), also largely collagenous, is posterior to the anterior limiting lamina. Transmission electron micrograph of monkey. Magnification: ×2,800.

lactic acid dehydrogenase (an enzyme that converts pyruvic acid to lactic acid during anaerobic metabolism). Both changes are presumably related to corneal hypoxia (Smelser and Ozanics 1952; Uniacke and Hill 1972). Metabolically required glucose and amino acids are believed to be transported into the cornea from the aqueous humor (Hale and Maurice 1969: Riley 1977).

Rapid regeneration of the epithelium occurs after wounding. Healing occurs by a combination of cell sliding and mitosis. If the entire epithelium is removed,

Table 6.1   Chemical Composition of the Corneal Stroma*

	%
Water	78
Collagen	15
Other proteins	5
Keratan sulfates	0.7
Chondroitin sulfates	0.3
Salts	1

*After Maurice DM (1969): The cornea and the sclera. In Davson H (ed.): The Eye, Vol. 1. New York, Academica Press.

the epithelial basement membrane may be recovered within a few days by a one-cell thick layer generated from the limbal conjunctiva. Several weeks may be required to reestablish the normal cellular pattern and biochemistry. Smaller wounds heal primarily by the sliding of cells, principally wing cells, and probably in a centripetal fashion.

The *anterior limiting lamina,* or *Bowman's membrane,* is a portion of the underlying stroma that is about 5 to 6 μm thick. This tissue exists in few vertebrates besides primates and in some birds and reptiles. It is acellular, being composed entirely of very fine collagen fibers and ground substance. Its anterior surface is distinct, but its posterior aspect blends into the stroma.

The *stroma* (also called the *substantia propria*) is the major structural component of the cornea, composing 90% of its thickness. The stroma provides strength, elasticity, and form to the cornea. The chemical composition of the stroma is given in Table 6.1; collagen (primarily type I, although variable amounts of other collagens, including types III and IV, have also been reported), other proteins, and glycosaminoglycans (GAGs) (principally keratan and chondroitin sulfates) are important fractions. GAGs make up 4.5% of the dry weight of the stroma in contrast to about 1% of the dry weight of the sclera. The importance of this particular difference will become apparent when the properties of the two tissues are compared.

The stroma contains several hundred organized bundles of parallel collagen fibrils called *lamellae,* each about 2 μm thick, 0.25 to 2 to 3 mm wide, and running from limbus to limbus but crossing at approximately right angles (Figure 6.3). Lamellae vary in size, sometimes dividing and rejoining; some interweaving may occur, consistent with the tendency of the lamellae to form waves when the cornea is distorted (Maurice and Monroe 1990). Although the stroma can support high tensile forces (an isolated and mounted cornea can withstand a fluid pressure of 30 atmospheres), it has little resistance to shearing forces. The lamellar layers of the stroma slide over each other very easily, as can be confirmed by holding this tissue between thumb and forefinger and moving the two faces relative to each other. Also, a blunt surgical dissecting instrument is known to

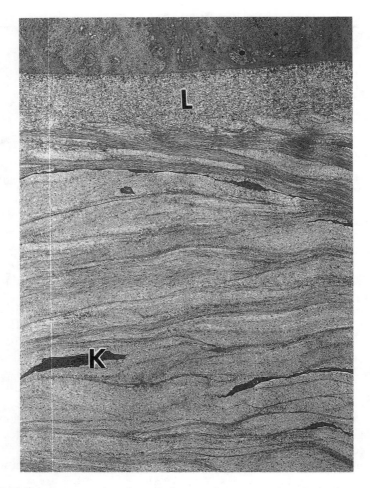

Figure 6.3A Transverse section through the anterior stroma. Anteriorly the stroma is continuous with the anterior limiting lamina (*L*). In contrast to the anterior limiting lamina, the collagen in the stroma is organized into distinct lamellae. These lamellae show less regularity anteriorly, being thinner, more undulating, and more intertwined than their posterior counterparts. Unlike the anterior limiting lamina the stroma contains keratocytes (*K*). Transmission electron micrograph of monkey. Magnification: ×2,800.

easily slide within a plane in the corneal stroma during a surgical corneal lamellar grafting procedure.

The collagen fibrils are of relatively uniform diameter (about 20 to 30 μm) within the lamellae. The center-to-center spacing also appears uniform at about 60 nm. Each fibril has a band at intervals of 21 nm along its length, with every third band more marked to give the 64-nm banding pattern of typical collagen.

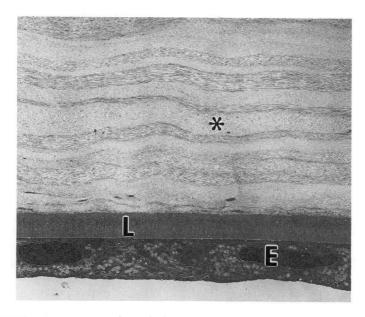

Figure 6.3B Transverse section through the posterior cornea. The lamellae forming the posterior stroma (*asterisk*) are uniform and are laid down flat on top of each other without intertwining. Posteriorly the stroma is lined by the posterior limiting lamina (*L*), which is the basement membrane of the endothelium (*E*). Transmission electron micrograph of monkey. Magnification: ×2,800.

The size and banding of these fibrils suggest, by comparison with collagen in other tissues, that this is embryonic collagen, having remained in an immature state since its production.

The ground substance surrounding and coating the collagen fibrils, mostly GAGs, fills all the space not occupied by these fibrils, the rare stromal cells, or nerves. The ground substance is highly hydrophilic (water-loving), and this property is responsible for the high water content of the stroma and thereby the phenomenon of swelling pressure (see later).

The stroma contains some cells (estimated from electron micrographs to be 3% to 5% by volume); these are mostly fibroblasts (known as *keratocytes*), which are believed to reside principally between rather than within the lamellae. These flat, spindle-shaped cells have large nuclei and long, thin, branching processes that appear to almost touch each other. The normal metabolic activities of the keratocytes appear similar to other corneal cells when judged by measured oxygen uptake rates.

Under certain inflammatory conditions, clusters of leukocytes, which have migrated from the limbal arcades via the tears or perhaps from the anterior chamber, become observable in the biomicroscope as corneal "infiltrates" (usually around the level of Bowman's membrane).

Wounds into and through Bowman's layer and then into the stroma typically heal with some irregularity, leading to opacification. There is an immediate swelling of the tissue, while local keratocytes take on the appearance and attributes of fibroblasts. Polymorphonuclear leukocytes (PMNs) and monocytes reach the wound site during the immediate inflammatory phase; the latter may also begin to look and act like fibroblasts. Epithelial cells may eventually fill the healing wound up to the corneal surface, to be gradually replaced by collagen laid down by the fibroblasts; eventually the epithelial plug is forced upward as strengthening and remodeling of the maturing wound occur over the course of weeks to years; some corneal wounds may never totally "heal."

The *posterior limiting lamina,* or *Descemet's membrane,* is the basement membrane of the endothelial cell layer. This membrane thickens throughout life from about 5 μm to greater than 10 μm, due to its continuous secretion by the endothelial cells. It is strong and partially elastic, composed of collagenous filaments and glycoproteins (including fibronectin), and it is periodic acid–Schiff (PAS) positive. When viewed by transmission electron microscope, normal Descemet's membrane consists of both a 3-μm thick anterior banded layer (formed prior to birth) and a thicker posterior homogeneous nonbanded layer that grows throughout life (Waring et al. 1982). Periodic excrescences or thickenings of Descemet's membrane may be observed in the periphery of normal adult human corneas; these dome-shaped areas are covered with altered endothelial cells and are known as *Hassall-Henle warts.* Measurements of the resistance to water flow through Descemet's membrane indicate that this tissue is more dense than the stroma (see below).

Ruptures of Descemet's membrane are clinically noted by parallel-sided linear gaps in this tissue; such damage may occur in buphthalmos, contusions and compressive trauma to the globe, and most commonly birth trauma (i.e., forceps delivery). The edges of such gaps curl posteriorly, demonstrating the tissue's elasticity. In time, if the endothelium is sufficiently young, these edges may be covered and additional Descemet's membrane will be laid down on top.

The endothelial cells line the anterior chamber side of the cornea (Figure 6.4). These cells are about 20 μm wide and 4 to 5 μm thick in humans and normally form a mosaic surface of polygonal (primarily hexagonal) cells in a monolayer. Aging and disease can disturb this surface pattern, decreasing the cell population below the normal 2000 to 3000/mm² (Yee et al. 1985), apparently creating cells of abnormally large or small surface areas (polymegethism) and changing cell shape (pleomorphism). Contact lens wear, where oxygen supply is known to be restricted, is also associated with similar changes in endothelial cell shape and size (Schoessler 1987) (Figure 6.5). Clinical observation of a decrease in cell number below 500 to 1000 cells/mm² is believed to be an indication of possible imminent corneal decompensation.

The endothelial cells have large oval and kidney-shaped nuclei, and they contain large numbers of organelles, including mitochondria, Golgi apparatus, and rough endoplasmic reticulum. The cell membrane has pinocytotic vesicles on both anterior and posterior sides; the latter shows about 20 to 30 microvilli per

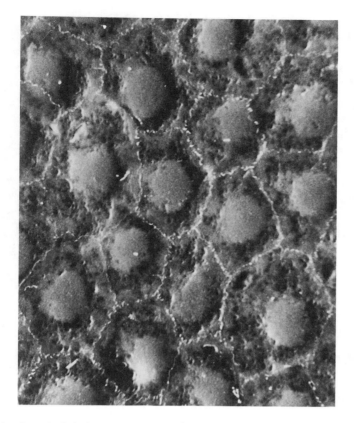

Figure 6.4 *A,* endothelial mosaic in young human. Microvilli demarcate the outline of the endothelial cells, which do not vary greatly in size. Note that five- and seven-sided cells are present together with the more common hexagons. The nucleus is represented by an elevation of the cytoplasm, but this may be artifactual. Scanning electron micrograph of 4-year-old human with no history of contact lens wear. Magnification: ×600.

cell, each measuring 0.1 to 0.2 μm wide and 0.5 to 0.6 μm high (Hogan et al. 1971). The lateral membranes between the endothelial cells have somewhat tortuous courses, separating cells by an overall space about 20 nm in width (see Figure 6.4B). Cells are joined, however, in various places by zonulae occludentes (most often in the more posterior third of the cell, closer to the anterior chamber side), as well as by maculae occludentes and rare maculae adherentes. Pleomorphism may stretch these membranes into a less convoluted but more oblique course (Figure 6.6) (Bergmanson 1990). Mitoses may be seen in the young human endothelium and in certain animals but is believed to be extremely rare in adult human cornea.

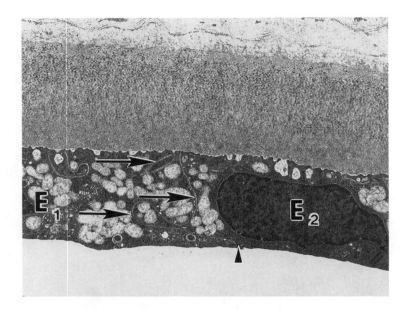

Figure 6.4 *B,* transverse section through the endothelium. The junction (*arrows*) between two endothelial cells (*E1, E2*) demonstrates extensive interdigitations, but its overall orientation remains approximately vertical. A zonula occludens (*triangle*) along the posterior border prevents aqueous from gaining free access to the endothelium and stroma. Transmission electron micrograph of 4-year-old human with no history of contact lens wear. Magnification: ×12,000. (Published with the permission of Bergmanson JPG [1991]: Histopathological analysis of corneal endothelial polymegathism. Cornea, in press.)

The endothelium, in particular the lateral space between the cells, is known to be the site of an ATPase-mediated active transport process that maintains stromal hydration (Maurice 1972; Hodson 1977) and secondarily clarity. A force generated by the "swelling pressure" of the stromal ground substance acts in the direction that would draw water into the stroma across both cellular boundary layers (epithelium and endothelium). A force generated by an osmotically active ion, probably bicarbonate, at the posterior surface of the endothelium, however, acts in the direction opposite to the swelling pressure so that there is no net force driving water into or out of the normal cornea under steady-state conditions. These osmotically active ions are deposited on the posterior surface of the endothelium by the metabolically driven process in the endothelial cells. It is this equilibrium of water-driving forces that maintains stromal hydration at a level at which the corneal stroma is transparent. These concepts will be discussed in detail in Chapter 7.

Damage to the corneal endothelium, either by disease (i.e., Fuchs dystrophy) or injury, may lead to stromal and epithelial swelling and reduced adhesion of the

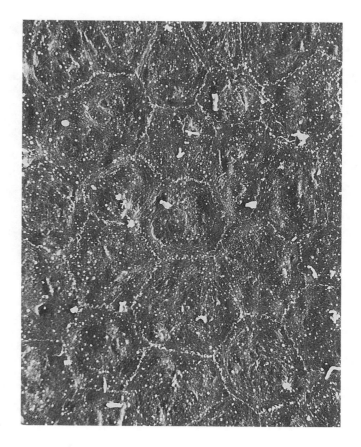

Figure 6.5 Endothelial mosaic of contact lens wearer. Polymegathism and polygonality are marked. Scanning electron micrograph of 66-year-old human who wore daily-wear aphakic soft lens correction for 13 years. Magnification: ×600. (Published with the permission of Bergmanson JPG [1991]: Histopathological analysis of corneal endothelial polymegathism. Cornea, in press.)

epithelial layer. Fluid retention between epithelial cells is called *microcystic edema* if mild but can lead to *bullous keratopathy* if severe. Corneal decompensation and decreased vision may follow.

SWELLING PRESSURE

Swelling pressure is the "keystone" of corneal biophysics, as it links stromal hydration and thickness and also affects corneal transparency through control of the anatomical separation of stromal collagen fibrils.

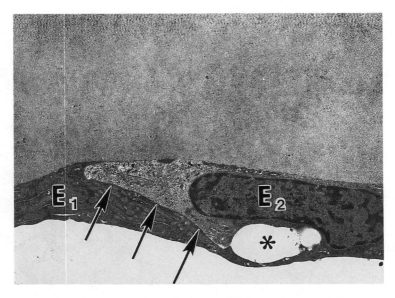

Figure 6.6 Transverse section through the endothelium of a contact lens wearer. The junction (*arrows*) between two neighboring cells (*E1, E2*) lacks interdigitations and has an oblique orientation. Corneal stress has led to the formation of an edematous space (*asterisk*) between the cells. Transmission electron micrograph of a 66-year-old human who wore daily-wear aphakic soft contact lens correction for 13 years. Magnification: ×12,000. (Published with the permission of Bergmanson JPG [1991]: Histopathological analysis of corneal endothelial polymegathism. Cornea, in press.)

The swelling pressure of the corneal stroma can be demonstrated by placing a piece of this tissue between two porous plates, submerged in water to avoid drying effects, and then using a weight on the upper plate to provide a constant force to squeeze the tissue (see Figure 6.7). A sample stroma, at equilibrium, will take on a fixed and unique water content (or hydration) for each level of such force. The same result is found if a whole cornea is used, but more time is needed to reach each new equilibrium water content when the weight is changed; we will later see that the epithelium and endothelium have a high resistance to water flow and this slows down the movement of water in and out of the stroma in response to the change in the weight.

The weight in Figure 6.7 imposes an inwardly directed force on the tissue. At equilibrium this force must be balanced by an outwardly directed force of the same magnitude, because it is only when the two forces are equal that the tissue will stop being further thinned. The outwardly directed force within this tissue is provided by the GAG ground substance between the collagen fibers, principally by negatively charged groups on the GAGs that repel one another. Further evidence supporting the thesis that the GAGs are the source of the swelling pressure comes from the observation that treatment of the stroma with cetyl pyridinium chloride,

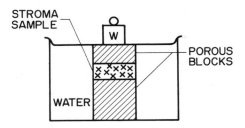

Figure 6.7 Stroma sample being subjected to a mechanical load W (the upper porous block is assumed to have no weight) to give, at equilibrium, a swelling pressure W/A, where A is the area of the sample.

known to precipitate GAG, causes its collapse; a cornea treated with cetyl pyridinium chloride will lose almost all of its water at a very low mechanical load.

The swelling force is largely perpendicular to the corneal surface because the collagen fibrils resist any change in the length of the lamellae. This effect is vividly demonstrated if a disk of mammalian stroma (perhaps 6 mm in diameter) is placed in water. Under this free-swelling condition, the tissue (normally about 0.4 mm thick) will swell to 10 to 30 times its normal thickness without much change in diameter. *In vivo*, a rabbit cornea will swell to about twice its normal thickness if the epithelium is removed but even more if the endothelium is destroyed (Maurice and Giardini 1951).

The mechanical load or weight per unit area required to maintain a submerged tissue slab at a fixed water content is called the *swelling pressure* of this tissue. Stromal swelling pressure at normal hydration and thickness is usually about 80 gm/cm^2 (Maurice 1969), which is equivalent to 60 mmHg.

Water content is usually expressed in grams of water per gram of dry material and is called *hydration*. Normal stromal hydration is about 3.5 gm water/gm dry material. The amount of dry material in a given piece of swelling tissue, however, may be difficult to determine. Easily diffusible substances, such as salts, may leave a tissue in varying amounts when it is submerged in a swelling pressure test. Prolonged soaking may also cause loss of some of the large organic constituents.

The swelling pressure versus hydration curve for corneal stroma is usually obtained by measuring the hydration of a tissue sample in an ascending staircase of progressively greater mechanical loads. Hydration should be a unique function of swelling pressure and should be independent of the history of the material. Experimentally, however, a hysteresis in the swelling pressure–hydration relationship is often noted. If, at some point, the load is *reduced*, water or aqueous solution is imbibed, but the new point found on the swelling pressure curve will be below the previously acquired data. Therefore, a swelling pressure curve obtained by increasing the load on the tissue sample is not reproduced when the load is removed. This hysteresis phenomenon is clearly demonstrated by continually loading and unloading a corneal sample between two fixed swelling pressures;

each successive change causes a smaller change in hydration of the sample. The direction of this change in the curves suggests that there is a loss of GAGs during acquisition of the initial data. Hara and Maurice (1972) observed GAGs in the solution leaving a sample tissue when a load was applied, so with continual reversals of load there might be significant loss of GAGs. Both experimental data (Kangas et al. 1988) and clinical observations (Holden et al. 1985) suggest this might also occur *in vivo*, as some forms of corneal edema have been found to result in long-term corneal thinning.

Bert and Fatt (1970) suggested that only the swelling components of a sample should be considered when studying swelling pressure as a function of hydration, as the inert materials in the sample occupy only volume. In the corneal stroma, for example, they recommend that hydration be defined as grams of water per gram of GAG, as the collagen fibrils provide only an inert meshwork that holds these GAGs. This proposal has not, however, been universally adopted.

Swelling pressure can also be theoretically related to the vapor pressure of water in a gas surrounding an excised swelling tissue. The amount that the stroma lowers the water vapor pressure below that of pure water, however, is too small to be easily measured. *In vitro* swelling pressure measurements are there-fore usually made on stroma samples by some variation of the process shown in Figure 6.7, in which a mechanical load is applied to compress a sample under water. *In vivo* measurements are based on somewhat different principles, to be described later.

The swelling pressure–hydration relationship for corneal stroma appears to be the same in human, rabbit, and steer samples, as shown in Figure 6.8. This relationship also appears to be almost independent of the salt concentration in the solution surrounding the tissue; Figure 6.8 shows similar swelling pressure data for rabbit stroma in pure water, isotonic saline (i.e., 1% NaCl), and 10% NaCl solution. Only a slight change in hydration is observed in comparing the results of tissue soaked in distilled water or 10% NaCl solution at a given swelling pressure. This is expected, since the salt provides positive ions that can gather around the negatively charged GAG molecules to shield some of the charges from each other and reduce the repulsion force discussed earlier—and leads to the noted slight decrease in hydration for the same swelling pressure. The near independence of stromal swelling pressure to the salt content of the surrounding fluid, however, is an indication that stromal swelling is not a simple osmotic phenomenon as might be observed on whole cells (red blood cells, for example, swell in hypotonic solutions). The stroma is not semipermeable, particularly to small ions such as Na^+ or Cl^-, in contrast to the red blood cell outer membrane.

Hedbys and Dohlman (1963) observed that the swelling pressure (P) verses hydration (H) relationship could be expressed by the equation

$$P = ae^{-bH} \qquad (6.1)$$

where a and b are constants. Equation 6.1 will yield a straight line when the data are plotted on semilogarithmic coordinates as shown in Figure 6.9. The equation of the straight line is $\log_e P = \log a - bH$.

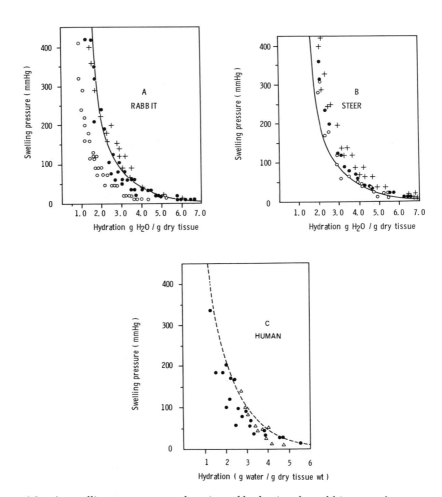

Figure 6.8 *A*, swelling pressure as a function of hydration for rabbit corneal stroma. Data taken in the direction of decreasing hydration. +, distilled water; •, 1% NaCl; ○, 10% NaCl; ——, from Hedbys and Dohlman (1963). *B*, swelling pressure as a function of hydration for steer corneal stroma. Data taken in the direction of decreasing hydration. +, distilled water; •, 1% NaCl; ○, 10% NaCl; ——, from Hedbys and Dohlman (1963). *C*, swelling pressures as a function of hydration for human stroma at 25°C. Data for • from Fatt and Hedbys (1970a), data for Δ from Hedbys and Dohlman (1963); ---, least squares line fitted to rabbit as logarithm of swelling pressure versus hydration.

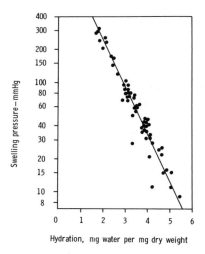

Figure 6.9 Swelling pressure as a function of hydration for steer stroma. The experimental data from Hedbys and Dohlman (1963) have been plotted on a semi-logarithmic graph.

When the swelling pressure of a disk of stroma submerged in water is balanced by a mechanical load, the system is at equilibrium and there is no tendency for water to move in or out of the tissue (Figure 6.10). If the load is increased, water will move out of the stroma because the water pressure inside the tissue has temporarily become greater than the outside pressure. Conversely, if the load is decreased, water will move in because the internal water pressure is temporarily lower than the outside water pressure. If the water surrounding the tissue is at atmospheric pressure, as it would be in an open vessel, then a negative pressure (with respect to the atmosphere) would be temporarily created inside the stroma by removing the load. Differences in pressure between the water inside and outside the sample stroma created when the load is changed will disappear as water moves in or out of the sample.

If the water surrounding the *in vitro* stroma sample in Figure 6.10 is removed *before* reducing the load, then a permanent negative water pressure could be created within the tissue on this reduction. This negative pressure is called the *imbibition pressure*. For any given hydration, the imbibition pressure is equal in magnitude but opposite in sign to the swelling pressure.

In the living eye, the collagen fibrils are also under a tensile stress caused by intraocular pressure (IOP). The fibrils are completely surrounded by a GAG gel that cannot transmit a shearing force. These fibrils can, however, exert a compressive force on the gel, and this force can be transmitted from one fibril to another. Because the outermost layer of fibrils has no layer above it, it has a minimum compressive force on it. Each underlying layer is then subject to the sum of all the compressive forces produced by the layers above it. The system is analogous to a

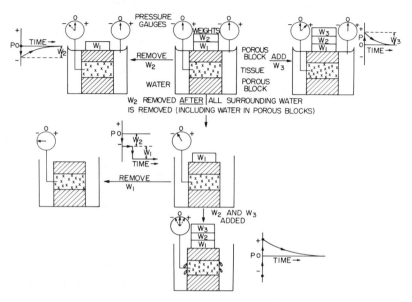

Figure 6.10 Relationship of internal water pressure (left-hand pressure gauge connected to stroma sample) and mechanical load imposed upon sample. *Upper row center,* the sample is in equilibrium under a mechanical load of $W_1 + W_2$. ---> on the pressure gauges show the transient, instantaneous pressure condition when a weight is added or removed. Note that sample in the lower three drawings is surrounded by air.

pile of books: the top book has no weight on it, but the bottom book is compressed by the weight of all the books above it. Thus, in the absence of any other forces, the mechanical load on the stromal fibril layers would range from zero on the outer layer to a maximum equal to the IOP (about 17 mmHg) on the innermost layer.

The *in vivo* stroma, therefore, presents a slightly different situation than the *in vitro* stroma. The normal internal pressure (i.e., swelling pressure [*SP* in Equation 6.2] of 60 mmHg) is equal in magnitude to the imbibition pressure (*IP* in the equation), but the ratio of compressive load changes *in vivo* from outer to innermost layer. An imbibition pressure of −60 mmHg will give a compressive load on the outermost stromal fibril layer also of −60 mmHg, but imbibition pressure is reduced at the innermost layer by IOP:

$$IP = IOP - SP \tag{6.2}$$

(from Hedbys et al. 1963), or $IP = 17 - 60 = -43$ mmHg. The range of compressive load along a line normal to the corneal surface should be from 0 to 17 mmHg, and therefore internal stromal pressure changes from −60 to −43 mmHg. For the range of compressive load equivalent to this range of swelling pressures (see swelling pressure curves in Figure 6.8), the hydration range will be from 3.4 to 3.5 gm water/gm dry material. Fortunately, this is well within the range of hydration that allows stromal transparency, as will be seen when the optical properties of the stroma are discussed later.

SWELLING PRESSURE AND THE THICKNESS–HYDRATION RELATIONSHIP

The Maurice theory of stromal transparency (to be discussed in detail later) requires that the collagen fibrils of the stroma be arranged in a geometrically regular array with a center-to-center spacing of about 60 nm. Because there is a set number of collagen fibrils, this in turn indicates that there is a fixed stromal thickness to provide optimal transparency. An increase in stromal thickness would impart a wider than optimal spacing to the collagen fibrils; a decrease in stromal thickness would lead to a closer spacing; either could lead to a loss of transparency. Because of the nature of stromal tissue, it is unlikely that any material other than water or an aqueous solution could move in and out of the stroma to change its thickness. Thus, a specified stromal thickness is equivalent to a specified hydration of the tissue.

The relationship between thickness and hydration in the stroma is uniquely linear because water added to the stroma adds only to its thickness; there is little or no change in the surface area. The constancy of stromal surface area when water is added is a direct consequence of its structure; the collagen fibrils do not react with the water. Instead, the water content is held between the fibrils by the GAG gel. Additional water therefore simply swells the gel, and although the fibrils remain the same length, they are pushed apart.

Ehlers (1966) demonstrated that 1 volumetric unit of water added to the corneal stroma gives exactly 1 unit of increase in stromal volume; the volume of water and dry tissue can be directly added to give the total volume of wet tissue. There is no *a priori* reason to expect this strict additivity of water volume and dry tissue volume in the stroma. In fact, many water solutions of organic substances do not exhibit volume additivity. A mixture of 1 liter of ethyl alcohol and 1 liter of water, for example, yields only 1.8 liters of solution. But the observations of constancy of area and strict volume additivity in the cornea lead directly to a linear relationship between stromal thickness and hydration. Figure 6.11 shows this relation for rabbit, steer, rat, and human stroma.

Several interesting observations can be made from Figure 6.11:

1. Direct observation has shown that *in vivo* mammalian stroma has a hydration of about 3.5 gm water/gm dry material; the intercepts of all four lines at zero hydration (on the vertical axis) represent the thicknesses of dry materials. Figure 6.11 therefore leads to the conclusion that the difference in *in vivo* stromal thickness among several mammalian species is a direct consequence of differences in the amounts of dry tissue material.

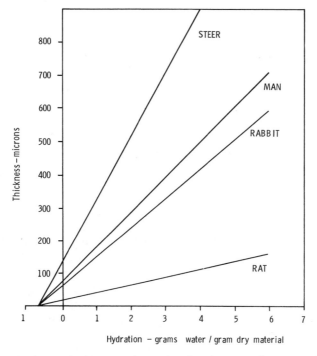

Figure 6.11 Thickness–hydration relationship for the corneal stroma of several mammals.

2. The common intercept of the four lines in Figure 6.11 at a zero thickness (at about −0.6 gm water/gm dry material of hydration) can be used to show that all species studied here have dry tissue of the same density (Hedbys and Mishima 1966). The numerical value of this intercept is the reciprocal of the dry tissue specific gravity (specific gravity is defined as the ratio of any material's density at 20°C to the density of water at 4°C).
3. Finally, Figure 6.11 can be used to explain the measured differences in human corneal thickness from center (0.52 mm) to limbus (0.65 mm). This difference must be ascribed to the stroma because the cellular layers (epithelium and endothelium) are far too thin to undergo the observed total thickness change. It is not yet possible to decide if this increase is due to greater hydration or greater amounts of GAG or because of a greater amount of total dry material.

It was previously shown that a difference in swelling pressure causes a flow of water (see Figure 6.10). Water moves from a point of lower swelling pressure to a point of higher swelling pressure. Another example of this is shown in Figure 6.12. Two halves of a strip of stroma are clamped to different thickness values and allowed to come to equilibrium in moist air or under oil. The clamps are then

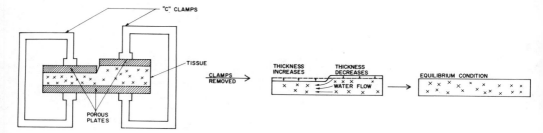

Figure 6.12 Demonstration of water movement from zone of higher hydration to zone of lower hydration.

removed. The water in the thicker portion (at a higher hydration and lower swelling pressure) must then move to the thinner part (lower hydration and higher swelling pressure) until the strip is again of uniform thickness. Hedbys and Mishima (1966) found this to be quite a slow process, suggesting high resistance to water flow across the cornea, consistent with clinical observations of dellen* where dehydration of a portion of corneal surface is not rapidly compensated by a lateral movement of water from the adjacent stroma. But, when equilibrium (no-flow condition) is again established, all portions of the normal stroma should be at about the same hydration and swelling pressure.

If the stroma is made of uniform material, it should have a similar hydration and thickness at all points in the absence of water flow along the stroma; yet if we accept that the cellular layers (epithelium and endothelium) are relatively uniform in thickness across the corneal surface and together sum to about 60 μm of thickness, by subtraction from values for corneal thickness given above, we expect the central human stroma to be 460 μm thick and the limbal portion to be 610 μm thick. Use of Figure 6.11 would suggest this thickness difference reflects a difference in stromal hydration from the central to the limbal region of 3.5 to 5.0 gm water/gm dry weight, respectively. Figure 6.8 converts these hydration values to swelling pressures to indicate that the center of the stroma is at a swelling pressure of 40 mmHg, whereas the limbus is at 25 mmHg. A study by Wiig (1989) provides data from the corneas of several mammalian species (including humans) supporting such a hypothesis. This pressure difference would predict an inwardly directed radial flow of water in the stroma of about 0.03 μl/hour. If this in fact exists, it represents only a small movement of water compared to the flow expected across the stroma from the aqueous to the tears.

An alternative explanation, however, is that there is no difference in hydration between the central and limbal regions, but that there is a difference in the amount of dry material. The known change in radius of curvature at the limbus (see the discussion of stress distribution in Chapter 8) also would suggest a need for additional structural support in this area.

*Dellen are depressions observed on the surface of the cornea. The epithelium in the depression is normal so the depression is considered to be an area in which the stroma has thinned.

It also appears that the anterior and posterior stroma may have slightly differing characteristics, both in terms of optical properties (some difference is apparent even in scattering within an optical section observed by biomicroscopy) and in water absorption. The anterior portion of the stroma has been found to imbibe less water than its posterior (Kikkawa and Hirayama 1970; Castoro et al. 1988), suggesting both a lower hydration and increased swelling pressure there. This might be related to a greater amount of keratin sulfate (compared to chondroitin sulfate) in the posterior stroma (Bettelheim and Goetz 1976; Castoro et al. 1988) or to some interweaving of the lamellae.

IN VIVO MEASUREMENT OF SWELLING–IMBIBITION PRESSURE

In vivo measurement always determines imbibition pressure as a function of stromal thickness. Figure 6.13 shows the procedure described by Hedbys, Mishima, and Maurice (1963). A fine plastic tube was implanted in the central region of the stroma of an anesthetized living rabbit. After the initial trauma of the procedure had subsided, the water-filled tube was connected to a pressure transducer, as shown in Figure 6.13, and water suction was measured. An optical pachometer, similar to that shown in Figure 6.14, was used to monitor corneal thickness. Alternatively, Klyce, Dohlman, and Tolpin (1971) inserted a disk of hydrophilic plastic (whose swelling pressure versus thickness relationship was known) into the stroma. They measured the thickness of this plastic disk within the stroma optically after healing. As discussed above, at equilibrium the imbibition pressure should be about the same at all points in both the stroma and the plastic, so that the stromal imbibition pressure could be determined. Both groups found imbibition pressure at an expected value of about 50 mmHg.

TRANSPORT PROCESSES

The study of transport processes forms the core of modern biophysics. For a more detailed treatment than can be given here the reader is referred to texts on

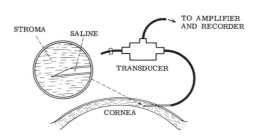

Figure 6.13 Schematic of the arrangement used to determine *in vivo* liquid pressure in the stroma. (From Hedbys BO, Mishima S, Maurice DM [1963]: The imbibition pressure of the corneal stroma. Exp. Eye Res. 2:99.)

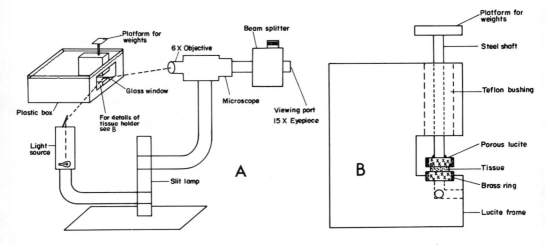

Figure 6.14 Schematic diagram of an optical apparatus used to measure tissue thickness as a function of applied mechanical load and of time. *A* shows a plastic box serving as a liquid bath for the pressure cell shown in *B*. The plastic box is fastened to the chin rest of a slitlamp. The microscope normally supplied with the slitlamp was replaced by one of high magnification (90×). The beam splitter replaced the eyepiece in one tube of the microscope. (With permission from Fatt I [1971]: Exp. Eye Res. 12:254. Copyright by Academic Press Inc. [London] Ltd.)

biophysics and physiology. It is unfortunate that the word *process* is used by the biologist for an anatomical feature and by the biophysicist for a physical and chemical mechanism. Here we will use the term to mean only the latter.

Before the advent of modern biophysics and the work of Katchalsky and Curran (1967), there was much confusion over two basic passive transport processes: *first,* the diffusion of dissolved species in a stationary solution, and *second,* the bulk flow of water—and the movement of dissolved substances carried along with this flow. Adding further complication, in biological tissues such as the eye, diffusion and bulk flow occur in water-bearing matrices and not in simple water solutions. Also, active transport, perhaps against a concentration gradient, is a potential *third* mechanism that is often observed in biological tissues such as the eye (see Chapter 2).

Theory of Diffusion

First we will discuss *diffusion*. In Figure 6.15, a tissue membrane separates a water solution of substance *A* in chamber 1 from another chamber (chamber 2) containing pure water. Let us start with a membrane saturated with water but free of solute *A*. Immediately on bringing the two chambers up to the membrane, solute *A* will begin to diffuse into the membrane, finally emerging from the membrane into chamber 2 containing pure water. We will also assume that the

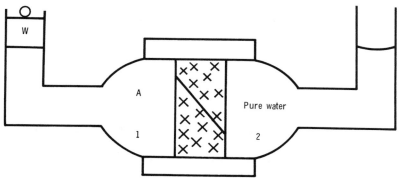

Figure 6.15 Schematic drawing of a cell in which only diffusion can take place. *Left,* chamber 1 contains a solution of concentration. *A*; *right,* chamber 2 contains pure water. The weight *W* provides a pressure to chamber 1 that balances any osmotic pressure that could cause flow of water from right to left. There is a concentration gradient in the porous membrane separating chamber 1 from chamber 2. The condition shown in the drawing exists only for an instant after the solution and pure water are put into their chambers.

two chambers are kept at or very close to their initial conditions by continuously passing solution *A* through chamber 1 and fresh water through chamber 2.

We immediately note that even though the membrane passes solute, we are maintaining a concentration difference across the membrane. Such concentration differences, as previously shown, can create an osmotic pressure difference and an accompanying flow of water, in this case from chamber 2 to chamber 1. To avoid, for the moment, the complication of water movement counter to the direction of diffusion, we will also postulate that the membrane is so resistant to water flow that such flow is negligible in this instance—or we could impose a hydrostatic pressure on chamber 1 equal in magnitude but opposite in sign to the osmotic pressure to counter any osmotic driving force appearing in the water in chamber 2.

Having established a situation where there will be no flow of water into the membrane, we can examine simple diffusion of substance *A* through the membrane. The movement will be from left to right, and the amount of *A* moved per unit time at the steady state will be given by an expression of Fick's law,

$$J = \frac{dm}{dt} = D_e \, a \frac{C}{L} \tag{6.3}$$

where *J* is the mass of *A* moving per unit time (dm/dt), and *a* is the area of the membrane and *L* its thickness. *C* is the mass concentration of *A* in the membrane at its left-hand surface (concentration here is in grams per cubic centimeter) and D_e is a proportionality constant called the diffusion coefficient. In this case, D_e depends on the properties of substance *A* and the membrane material. In the more general case (where there is some *A* at both surfaces at all times) Equation 6.3 becomes

$$J = \frac{dm}{dt} = D_e \, a\frac{\Delta C}{L} \tag{6.4}$$

where ΔC is the difference in concentration of A across the membrane. In more advanced treatments, Fick's law is usually written as

$$j = \frac{J}{a} = -D_e \frac{dC}{dx} \tag{6.5}$$

where j is the value of dm/dt per unit area. The negative sign before the D_e signifies that the movement of A is down the concentration gradient dC/dx in the x direction.

From a dimensional analysis of Equation 6.4, we can write

$$\frac{gm}{sec} = D_e \; (cm^2) \left(\frac{[gm/cm^3]}{cm}\right) \tag{6.6}$$

Thus, to give the same dimensions on both sides, D_e must have the dimensions of cm^2/sec.

It must be emphasized that ΔC in Equation 6.4 refers to the solute concentration difference between points *just inside* the outer surfaces, or *boundaries,* of the membrane. This means that ΔC is *not* the difference in solute concentrations between the chambers on opposite sides of the membrane. Very often, however, only the solute concentrations in the chambers are known and there is usually a fixed ratio between the solute concentrations in the chambers and the concentration inside the immediately adjacent boundaries within the membrane. The solute concentration in the membrane surface in contact with chamber 1 in Figure 6.15 can be written as

$$C_{m1} = k_s \, C_{c1} \tag{6.7}$$

where C_{m1} is the concentration in the membrane surface, C_{c1} is the concentration in chamber 1, and k_s is a constant called the *partition coefficient.* For the other side of the membrane, similarly

$$C_{m2} = k_s \, C_{c2} \tag{6.8}$$

If Equation 6.8 is subtracted from Equation 6.7, the ΔC term for Equation 6.4 becomes

$$\Delta C = C_{m2} - C_{m1} = k_s \, (C_{c2} - C_{c1}) = k_s \, \Delta C_c \tag{6.9}$$

Inserting this result into Equation 6.4 gives

$$\frac{dm}{dt} = D_e \, k_s \, a\frac{\Delta C_c}{L} \tag{6.10}$$

In many biological systems the thickness of the membrane is not known or measurable. Biologists therefore have used the group $D_e k_s/L$ to express the amount of material diffusing through a unit area of membrane of unknown thickness when the difference in solute concentration between the opposite chambers is ΔC_c. In the biological literature this group is called the *permeability*.

In the contact lens literature, however, Dk is considered *permeability*, and when lens thickness (which is usually known or measurable and identified as L) is included, the term Dk/L is called *transmissibility*. This will be discussed in Chapter 7.

It is of interest now to examine some of the factors that control the magnitude of D_e. For example, D_e is affected by the nature of the *solute* (e.g., the *size*, or molecular weight, and the *shape* of its molecules), the nature of the *material* through which the diffusion occurs, and the *temperature*. We accept that a diffusing substance cannot penetrate the molecules of the tissue material but must move in the water phase of the wet tissue, passing around the molecules of tissue material. A large diffusing molecule will be slowed down for two reasons. It will have less velocity than a small molecule at any given temperature because of its larger mass, and the available thermal energy does not give as much motion to a heavy molecule as to a light molecule. Also, the large molecule must find large spaces through which to pass within the tissue material, and these spaces may be less frequent than smaller spaces. Interaction between the *electrostatic potentials* of both the diffusing species and the material through which diffusion is occurring, when present, is another factor that may play a role in the magnitude of D_e.

It is appropriate now to introduce the concept of *tension gradient*. In discussing the aqueous humor (Chapter 2), it was shown that the concentration of a gas dissolved in a liquid could be expressed as a tension. The relation of tension to dissolved gas concentration was shown to be given by Henry's law:

$$C = k\,P \qquad (6.11)$$

where k is similar to the partition coefficent but is called the *Henry's law constant* and is simply the *solubility* of gas per unit gas pressure (P). For convenience, when describing diffusion of a dissolved gas (e.g., oxygen, carbon dioxide) we will use concentration in terms of milliliters of gas, corrected to 0°C and 1 atm, dissolved in 1 ml of liquid or solid medium. Since biological tissues are largely composed of water, Henry's law can also be applied to them, noting that k may be somewhat smaller than for pure water. The solubility of the gas is then less on a volume-for-volume basis in tissue than in pure water.

If the expression for C in Equation 6.11 is substituted into Equation 6.4 (m is changed to v in milliliters for convenience)

$$J = \frac{dv}{dt} = D_e\,k\,a\,\frac{\Delta P}{L} \qquad (6.12)$$

Since k has the units of milliliters-gas/[(milliliter-tissue) × (units of gas tension)], Equation 6.12 will give the diffusion of gas in milliliters/time.

The importance of this discussion will become apparent when oxygen diffusion in both corneal tissues and contact lenses is examined in Chapter 7.

Theory of Bulk Flow

Now we will introduce another and different passive transport mechanism. If a tissue membrane (for our purposes here this will be the corneal stroma) is placed between two chambers, each of which is filled with pure water but to different heights, a hydrostatic pressure gradient of $\rho g h$ will occur, where ρ is the density of water, g is the acceleration due to gravity, and h is the difference in height between the liquid surfaces. This is illustrated in Figure 6.16, where the height of the water in the left-hand chamber is seen to be h above that of the water in the right-hand chamber. The rate of water movement from left to right through the membrane is given by *Darcy's law*, namely

$$\frac{dv}{dt} = \frac{k}{\mu} a \left(\frac{\rho g h}{L} \right) \tag{6.13}$$

where dv/dt is the volume flow of water per unit time, μ is the viscosity of the water, k is a constant that is a property of the membrane, and the other new terms are as defined immediately above.

This movement of water or aqueous solution through a membrane according to Darcy's law is called *convective* or *bulk flow*. As distinct from diffusion, where the solute molecules are moving individually and at random with a higher net rate in the direction down a *concentration* gradient than in any other direction, here water molecules are all moving in concert down a *pressure* gradient.

The difference in height of water in the left-hand chamber in Figure 6.16 is essentially an excess in force per unit area exerted on the left-hand side of the membrane compared to the right. Intensive study by biophysicists has shown that this hydrostatic force could be replaced by a force of another kind and the same result occurs. As examples, in Figure 6.17A the force is applied by gas pressure, and in Figure 6.17B the force is applied by a piston of weight W. If ΔP is the excess pressure applied to the water on one side, then Darcy's law is written in its more general form.

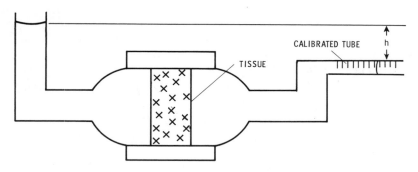

Figure 6.16 Schematic drawing of a cell in which a liquid is being forced to move through the tissue sample as a result of applying a driving force. $\rho g h$ where ρ is the liquid density, g the gravitational acceleration, and h the difference in height between source and sink.

$$\frac{dv}{dt} = \frac{k}{\mu} a \frac{\Delta P}{L} \qquad (6.14)$$

The term k/μ is the *flow conductivity* or *hydraulic conductivity* in biological literature because the viscosity is always that of water ($\mu = 1.0$ centipoise) and can be considered constant. Very often the thickness of the tissue or membrane is not easily measured or even defined. In those cases the term $k/\mu L$ is used to combine flow conductivity and thickness into a term called *flow conductance*. In engineering, where fluids of various viscosity are encountered, the k term in k/μ is treated separately and is called *permeability*.

From this discussion, and the above section on diffusion, it is apparent that biologists, engineers, and contact lens practitioners use the term *permeability* for different quantities; to add to confusion, permeability is also used as a magnetic property of a material in physics and electrical engineering. Confusion can be avoided by noting carefully the context in which the term is used and observing that biological permeability ($D_e k_s/L$) has the dimensions of length/time (usually centimeters per second), whereas engineering permeability has dimensions of

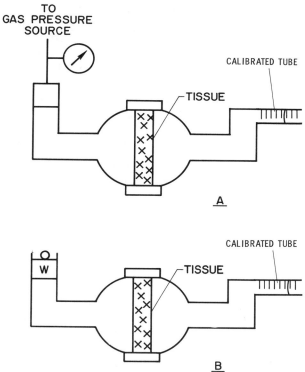

Figure 6.17 *A*, gas pressure is applied to free liquid surface to provide force that moves liquid through tissue sample. *B*, a moveable piston of weight *W* provides the force that moves the liquid through the tissue sample.

length squared (usually square centimeters but sometimes called the *Darcy;* the Darcy is 10^{-8} cm^2) and contact lens permeability (Dk) is in cm^{2}ml/sec ml mmHg.

As the flow rate predicted by Equation 6.14 is independent of the source of the pressure drop (ΔP), it is the same whether ΔP is an externally imposed pressure or a quantitatively equal osmotic pressure produced by a difference in solute concentration for a perfectly semipermeable membrane (one not penetrated by the solute). If the solute molecule can also enter the membrane (i.e., the membrane is *not* a perfectly semipermeable membrane), a detailed description of the system is beyond the scope of this book and the reader is referred to the text by Katchalsky and Curran (1967). For the purposes of this text, it is sufficient to note that if the solute gradient is in the same direction as the flow of water in the membrane, the rate of movement of solute is enhanced by the bulk flow of water. Conversely, if the solute concentration is in the opposite direction, water flow reduces solute movement through the membrane.

Stromal Diffusion

Maurice (1969) estimated the size of the spaces in the corneal stroma from an ingenious experiment. He injected a small amount of a solution of human hemoglobin into the center of a stroma at normal hydration. These molecules of hemoglobin (molecular weight about 68,000, diameter about 6.4 nm) were seen to diffuse away from the point of injection. He then repeated the experiment with larger hemoglobin from the mollusk *Planorbis* (with a molecular weight of about 1,630,000 and diameter of about 18.5 nm), and found that this molecule did not diffuse away from the injection site if the stroma was of normal hydration. If the stroma was allowed to imbibe water and swell to a hydration of 1.5 times its normal value, however, *Planorbis* hemoglobin began to diffuse within the stroma. Conversely, if normal stroma was dehydrated to 60% of its normal hydration, human hemoglobin no longer diffused within the tissue. Maurice concluded that spacing between the molecules in the normal stroma is about 12 nm. He further concluded that the diffusion of molecules within this tissue is controlled by the gel-like GAGs and not by the collagen fibers because these are spaced about 30 nm apart (center-to-center spacing of the collagen fibers is about 60 nm, but the fibers themselves occupy about half of this space). For later comparison, the reader should note that the size of the oxygen molecule (O_2, with a molecular weight of 32) is about 0.5 nm and fluorescein is about 1.1 nm.

Maurice (1969) also collected stromal diffusion data on a number of small substances. He showed that the diffusion coefficient of these small molecules in the normal stroma is only about 40% of the value found for the same molecules in pure water. This reduction is about the same along the tissue as across it, further supporting the hypothesis that it is the amorphous nonoriented gel between the fibrils rather than the fibrils themselves that determines resistance to diffusion.

Maurice and Watson (1965) studied the distribution and movement of serum albumin (about 7.5 nm in size) in the stroma and found that its naturally occurring concentration drops from the corneal periphery to the center. It was shown that this could be explained if it was assumed that this protein entered from the blood at the limbus and was lost across the corneal surfaces as it diffused (D_e of 1.2×10^{-7} cm^2/sec) toward the corneal center.

The immunoglobulin IgG measures about 12×3.5 nm (Maurice 1984) and has a molecular weight of about 140,000. Allansmith and co-workers (1979) and later Verhagen and colleagues (1990) found that IgG diffuses very slowly in corneal stroma ($D_e = 2.3 \times 10^{-8}$ cm^2/sec), and its free diffusion constant in water (D_e of 6.4×10^{-7} cm^2/sec at 37°C) indicates it is slowed by a factor of about 27 in the stroma.

Mondino and Brady (1981) studied the distribution in the cornea of the twenty or more serum proteins known collectively as *complement*. They found less complement in the central cornea compared to the periphery for all complements studied. The difference ratio was 1 to 5 for the largest component, with a molecular weight of 650,000. The ratio decreased to 1 to 1.2 for components with molecular weights near 120,000. These data suggest that diffusion of large molecules from the limbal vessels may bring these materials to the center of the cornea. Mondino and associates (1982) point out, however, that production of the high molecular weight components of complement by keratocytes in the cornea may explain its presence in the cornea. Wiig (1989, 1990) believes that bulk flow of water from the limbus to the center of the cornea may carry large molecules.

Bulk Flow in the Stroma

Hedbys and Mishima (1962) reported the flow conductance ($k/\mu L$) of steer stroma; they reported a value of about 5×10^{-11} cm^3/dyne sec for the normally hydrated tissue. The conductivity or k/μ was 1730×10^{-15} cm^4/dyne sec. Fatt and Hedbys (1970a) found similar results for human stroma. Flow conductivity of the stroma cannot be measured by simply placing this tissue between two chambers as shown in Figure 6.16. The unrestrained stroma would swell under these conditions, and the measured flow conductivity could not be related to any particular stromal thickness. The sample is instead placed between two porous plates that are positioned to maintain a fixed stromal thickness during measurement, and water flows through this combination. The flow resistance of the porous plates alone is determined by flowing water at a known pressure gradient through the assembly before the stroma is placed between them. The flow data obtained with the stroma in place may then be corrected for the resistance of the porous plates alone by using the well-known relation for resistances in series.

Fatt (1968a) used the apparatus shown in Figure 6.18 to measure flow conductivity of rabbit stroma by a transient method. This device applies a known mechanical load to an excised (i.e., *in vitro*) disk of corneal stroma while the equilibrium thickness of the tissue is monitored by electrical determination of plunger position. Fatt (1968a) produced the data seen in parts *A* and *B* of Figure

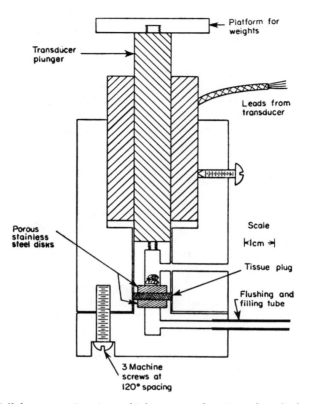

Figure 6.18 Cell for measuring tissue thickness as a function of applied mechanical load and of time. (With permission from Fatt I [1968]: Exp. Eye Res. 7:402. Copyright by Academic Press Inc. [London] Ltd.)

6.19, whereas part C is from Fatt and Hedbys (1970a). The pressure gradient required to move water through the stroma was provided by increasing the swelling pressure. It is clear from Figure 6.19 that flow conductivity of the stroma is strongly dependent on its hydration. As the water in the stroma is bound to the GAGs rather than to the collagen fibers, it appears that the hydration level of the GAGs determines the flow conductivity of the tissue.

Hedbys and Mishima (1962) found similar values for flow conductivity of steer stroma both perpendicular and parallel to the stromal surface. This observation provides additional evidence supporting the hypothesis that the resistance to water flow in the stroma is not provided by the fibers but by the amorphous gel substance between them. Maurice (1969) emphasized this point by showing that the engineering equation that predicts flow conductivity of fiber beds *fails* to predict the observed slow flow of water in the stroma when the GAG gel between the bed of collagen fibers is ignored.

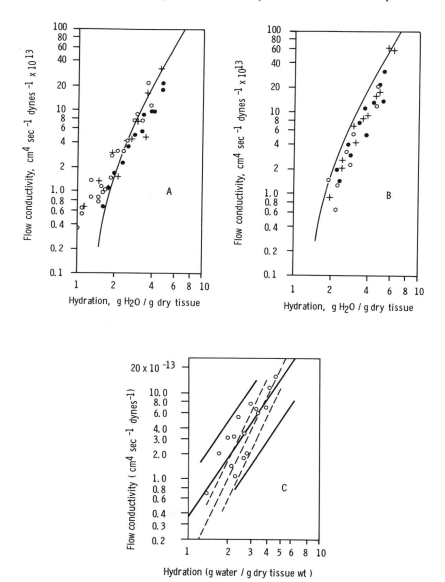

Figure 6.19 *A*, flow conductivity as a function of hydration for rabbit stroma at 25°C. +, distilled water; ●, 1% NaCl; o, 10% NaCl; ——, from Hedbys and Mishima (1962) for steer stroma. *B*, flow conductivity as a function of hydration for steer stroma at 25°C. +, distilled water; ●, 1% NaCl; o, 10% NaCl; ——, from Hedbys and Mishima (1962) for steer stroma. *C*, flow conductivity as a function of hydration for human stroma at 25°C. ——, fitted by least squares through human stroma data; ---, least squares line for rabbit stroma data. Outer lines represent 95% confidence limits.

The Limiting Layers

The limiting layers of the cornea, the epithelium and the endothelium, are important largely for the metabolic processes operating in their cells. These layers appear to adhere to the stroma in part because of the negative (swelling or imbibition) pressure in the stroma. If this negative pressure is overwhelmed by a high IOP as in acute glaucoma (recall Equation 6.2), for example (Figure 6.20), there may be a separation of portions of the epithelial cell layer from the underlying tissues, leading to a clinical condition called *bullous keratopathy* (Ytteborg and Dohlman 1965). Maurice (1984) also suggests that IOP is responsible, at least in part, for the adherence of the endothelium to Descemet's membrane.

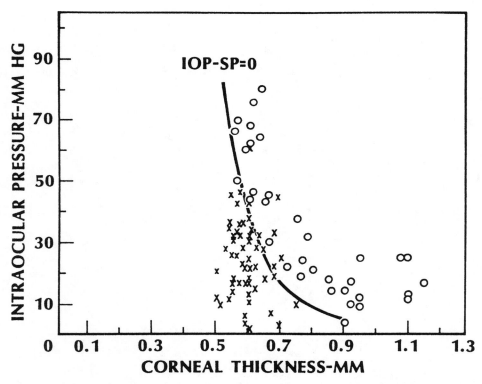

Figure 6.20 Thickness of cornea as a function of intraocular pressure in 90 human eyes. *Open circles* are for eyes with edema of the epithelial layer; *crosses* are for eyes without epithelial edema. The curve represents the swelling pressure–thickness relationship for corneal stroma. Fluid pressure would be expected to be positive in stromas represented by points to the right of the curve and negative for points to the left. (From Ytteborg J, Dohlman CH [1965]: Corneal edema and intraocular pressure. II. Clinical results. Arch. Ophthalmol. 74:477–484, with permission.)

The endothelium is a very fragile cellular layer and may be damaged or destroyed by simply touching it with a solid object, reducing its effectiveness as a physical barrier to water flow. Damage to the endothelium can occur during intraocular surgery, either due to surgical manipulation of the cornea, direct touch by an instrument or intraocular lens (IOL), or toxic effects of irrigating solutions.

The transport properties of the limiting layers have been studied extensively because these properties are very important to the nutrition of the cornea. Active transport and the passive transport of oxygen are specifically discussed in Chapter 7; here we present data for passive transport, both diffusion and bulk flow, in intact limiting layers.

Diffusion in the Limiting Layers

The *epithelium* has a low diffusion permeability $(D_e k_s/L)$ to ions and polar molecules. $D_e k_s/L$ has been found to be 0.8 to 2.5×10^{-7} cm/sec for the sodium ion (Maurice 1951; Maurice 1957a) and 0.4×10^{-8} cm/sec for fluorescein (an ion of a weak acid) (Maurice 1967). Maurice (1969) believes that ions (like Na^+, Cl^-, and fluorescein) can penetrate the intact epithelium only through its complex and tight intercellular channels. Resistance to such penetration is therefore quite high if the epithelial cells and their lateral junctions are intact. This phenomenon is the basis for the use of fluorescein in ocular surface examinations; if the epithelium is intact, a drop of fluorescein is soon washed off the corneal surface, but fluorescein penetrates the surface and stains the underlying layers if the epithelial surface is broken. Materials that are lipid soluble (nonpolar), however, such as alkaloids, steroids, and cholinesterase inhibitors, can penetrate the cornea in spite of their large molecular size. Such substances have a high solubility in the cell membrane (a high value of k_s); therefore, they can move quickly into the epithelial cells. The more recent work of Araie and Maurice (1987) supports these conclusions with additional data.

Most ophthalmic drugs are slightly ionized bases of the form R^+OH^-, where R^+ is an organic cation. The un-ionized molecule $R\,OH$ is lipid soluble and diffuses easily through the epithelial cell walls. A high concentration of un-ionized molecules favors an increased rate of penetration. Therefore, this kind of basic drug is usually applied to the eye in a solution high in OH^- concentration (high pH), so that the ionic equilibrium $R^+ + OH^- = R\,OH$ will be shifted to the right. Conversely, acidic drugs (such as salicylic acid) are applied in acid (or low pH) solution.

The penetration of water into and through the epithelium can be by either diffusion or bulk flow. Considering just diffusion for the moment, tracer studies using the deuterium (D) and tritium (T) isotopes of hydrogen (as D_2O and THO) for the diffusing species yield a value of 3×10^{-4} cm/sec for the $D_e k_s/_L$ of the epithelium. D_2O and THO are physically very similar to ordinary water and therefore are trace solutes of water-like molecules in solvent water. As we will see below, concentration gradients of water will cause an osmotic pressure difference that will induce a bulk flow of water that will transport much more water than is the case when diffusion is the transport mechanism.

Additionally, one must note that iontophoresis, which is the movement of ions (electrically charged molecules) into a tissue by means of a low-tension direct electrical current, has been used, at least experimentally, to accelerate the movement of material across the epithelium into the cornea (Jones and Maurice 1966; Bonnano and Polse 1987)

Maurice (1951, 1955) measured the diffusion of Na^+ through rabbit corneal *endothelium* and reported that $D_e k_s/L$ was equal to 2×10^{-5} cm/sec. Na^+ permeability of the endothelium is evidently 200 times larger than that of the epithelium. Permeability also decreases, as would be expected, with increasing size of the molecule; for example, the endothelial permeability to fluorescein is only about 3×10^{-6} (human) to 5×10^{-6} (rabbit) cm/sec (Ota et al. 1974). Ionic charge is believed to have only minor effects, if any, on diffusion in the endothelium. Such observations are important when one considers the behavior of topically applied pharmaceutical agents. Maurice (1969) found that placing a solution of small ions on the epithelial surface resulted in a corneal concentration of only 1% of that in the solution after a time of 2.5 to 3 hours (and reached only 1.1% at maximum). Diffusion into the aqueous will occur by this route but does not exceed 0.33% of the original precorneal concentration. Introducing the ion directly into the aqueous humor, on the other hand, produces a stable concentration in the whole cornea at some 80% of the aqueous concentration. Such observations show the relative inefficiency of drug solutions topically applied to the corneal surface compared to those that might be brought into the aqueous humor directly or indirectly.

Riley (1977) found that the permeability of the endothelium to three amino acids (glycine, aspartate, and alpha-aminoisobutyric acid) was equal in both aqueous-to-stroma and stroma-to-aqueous directions, and generally in the range expected for their size. Amino acids are needed to enable the epithelium to synthesize protein to replace that lost by the continual desquamation of surface cells. Riley concluded that diffusion across the endothelium and through the stroma supplies the cornea and most specifically the epithelium with the amino acids for metabolism; the permeability values found were consistent with the amount of protein required. Earlier observations of stromal concentrations in excess of aqueous humor concentrations were believed to be the result of accumulation of such amino acids in the stromal keratocytes.

Bulk Flow in the Limiting Layers

The flow conductivities of rabbit corneal epithelium and endothelium were individually measured by Mishima and Hedbys (1967). They used whole cornea as an osmometer, as shown in Figure 6.21, first with the epithelium being the semipermeable membrane and the stroma the internal vessel (into which water enters or leaves according to whether the external solution is less or more concen-

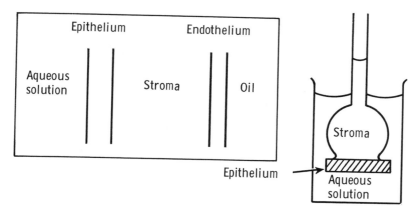

Figure 6.21 Model of the cornea acting as an osmometer. *Left,* the cornea; *right,* the equivalent osmometer.

trated than the internal solution). For this experiment the endothelial surface was blocked by application of a water-impermeable oil barrier. Although in practice their procedure required a more complicated analysis, in principle Darcy's law (Equation 6.14) was applied to the epithelium. The known solute concentration difference between the stroma and the outer solution gave the pressure drop via the osmotic pressure relationship: $\Delta P = \Delta C\,R\,T$. The rate of water flow across the epithelium was determined by noting the rate at which the stroma thickened or thinned. From the known thickness–hydration relationship of the stroma (see Figure 6.11), observed changes in thickness were interpreted as changes in hydration. Since the dry material in the stroma should remain constant during changes in hydration, it is clear that the observed change in thickness reflects movement of water into or out of the stroma. All of this water movement must take place across the epithelium because the endothelium is blocked by oil. Therefore, water flow across the epithelium was measured by observation of the rate of thickening or thinning of the stroma. Knowing the area and thickness of the epithelium in the sample under study, conductance $(k/\mu L)$ corrected for 35°C could be calculated and was found to be 0.7×10^{-11} cm³/dyne sec. If the epithelial layer thickness is taken as 39 μ, then conductivity (k/μ) becomes 27×10^{-15} cm⁴/dyne sec.

Similar study of the endothelium gave conductance at 1.55×10^{-11} cm³/dyne sec and conductivity as 7.8×10^{-15} cm⁴/dyne sec for a tissue layer 5 μm thick.

Recall that Hedbys and Mishima (1962) reported the flow conductance $(k/\mu L)$ of steer stroma as about 5×10^{-11} cm³/dyne sec (while conductivity was 1730×10^{-15} cm⁴/dyne sec for a tissue thickness of 350 μm). These data make intuitive sense because the epithelium and endothelium are cellular layers with lipid membranes and tight junctions between cells, whereas the stroma is a hydrophilic meshwork. Bowman's membrane should be very similar to stroma, which it resembles in tissue properties (see above), and also, as it is only about 10 μm thick, Bowman's membrane should have litte effect on the overall bulk flow of water.

Fatt (1969a) analyzed data from three earlier experiments (Maurice and Giardini 1951; Mishima and Hedbys 1967; Hara and Maurice 1969) and calculated the conductance $(k/\mu L)$ of Descemet's membrane to be 27×10^{-11} cm^3/dyne sec with a conductivity (k/μ) of 200×10^{-15} cm^4/dyne sec (this latter ranged from 111 to 280×10^{-15}). Descemet's membrane is thin and cannot offer much total resistance to overall corneal water flow.

Corneal Bulk Water Flow

Water flow conductivity data for the several layers of the cornea (Table 6.2) can now be used to estimate the movement of water by bulk flow across the whole tissue in the living eye. The cornea offers a total resistance to water flow that is the sum of resistance in series for each individual layer. Considering Bowman's membrane to be part of the stroma, which it closely resembles (and as it is very thin), we can treat the cornea as four layers in series, from inside the eye to the external surface: endothelium, Descemet's membrane, stroma, and epithelium. The law of resistance in series is

$$R_t = R_1 + R_2 + R_3 + R_4 \tag{6.15}$$

Table 6.2 Flow Conductivity of the Layers of the Cornea

	Endothelium	Descemet's Membrane	Stroma and Bowman's Membrane	Epithelium
k/μ (cm^4/dyne sec)	7.8×10^{-15}	200×10^{-15}	1730×10^{-15}	27×10^{-15}
Thickness (L in cm)	5×10^{-4}	10×10^{-4}	450×10^{-4}	50×10^{-4}
$k/\mu L$ (cm^3/dyne sec)	1.6×10^{-11}	20×10^{-11}	3.8×10^{-11}	0.5×10^{-11}
$\mu L/k$ (dyne sec/cm^3)	64×10^9	5×10^9	26×10^9	185×10^9
$R(= uL/ka)$ (dyne sec/cm^5)	49×10^9	3.9×10^9	20×10^9	142×10^9
R_t (dyne sec/cm^5)		215×10^9		
Fractional pressure drop	0.23	0.018	0.09	0.66

where R_t is total corneal resistance and R_1 to R_4 are the individual layer resistances. The flow resistance of any layer in the cornea is the reciprocal of its conductance over area (from Equation 6.14):

$$R = \left(\frac{\mu}{k}\right)\left(\frac{L}{a}\right) \qquad (6.16)$$

Therefore, the total flow resistance of the cornea (R_t) is

$$R_t = \left(\frac{\mu L}{ka}\right)_{en} + \left(\frac{\mu L}{ka}\right)_D + \left(\frac{\mu L}{ka}\right)_s + \left(\frac{\mu L}{ka}\right)_{ep}$$
$$= \left(\frac{\mu L}{ka}\right)_c \qquad (6.17)$$

From Darcy's law, the flow rate per unit area through the cornea is

$$\frac{dv}{dt} = \frac{\Delta P}{R_t} \qquad (6.18)$$

Table 6.2 gives the values used in the calculations above to determine R_t; k/μ values are from rabbit tissue, except for that of the stroma, which is from steer tissue. Thickness values were chosen to model the human cornea. Although these thicknesses are different from those of rabbit and steer, we believe these tissue properties, the k/μ values, are not much different for the different species. For this reason the $k\mu/L$ values given in Table 6.2 are considered good estimates for human cornea. Stanley (1972) indeed found similar data from *in vivo* studies on human corneas, but his data will not be used here because his measurements on the *in vivo* human eye seem less reliable due to experimental limitations necessary for the safety and comfort of his subjects.

From the values in Table 6.2 now corrected for human thicknesses, R_t is found to be 2.15×10^{11} dyne sec/cm^5. To use Equation 6.18, we must set a pressure drop (ΔP) across the cornea. When the eye is closed, the tear fluid can be assumed to be isotonic and therefore there is no osmotic pressure drop across the cornea. The pressure difference is solely IOP, which is normally about 18 mmHg, and as 1330 dyne/cm^2 = 1 mmHg, this represents 2.39×10^4 dyne/cm^2. Now Equation 6.18 gives

$$\frac{dv}{dt} = \frac{2.39 \times 10^4 \text{ dynes/cm}^2}{2.15 \times 10^{11} \text{ dynes sec/cm}^5}$$
$$= 1.11 \times 10^{-7} \frac{\text{cm}^3}{\text{sec}} \qquad (6.19)$$

Converted to microliters per minute, Equation 6.19 therefore shows that the possible flow through the cornea of the closed eye is only about 0.007 μl/min, and this represents only a very small part (perhaps 0.2%) of the total aqueous humor outflow.

When the eye is open, however, evaporation of water from the tear layer concentrates the aqueous component of the tears. Mishima and Maurice (1961a,b) found that normal open-eye tears are 10% more concentrated in salts than are fresh tears (which are isotonic). If the aqueous humor is assumed to be similar to an isotonic solution (equivalent to a 0.9% solution of sodium chloride), the open-eye cornea is separating this isotonic aqueous from the more concentrated tears (equivalent to about 1% sodium chloride). There is then a concentration difference of 35 millimoles/liter of dissolved species (sodium plus chloride ions) across the cornea. The osmotic pressure due to this difference is about 650 mmHg by Equation 2.1. The flow of water through the cornea from aqueous humor to tears caused by this osmotic pressure difference is about 0.28 μl/min. Since the total aqueous flow rate is about 2.5 μl/min (see Chapter 2), the outflow via the cornea of the open eye could represent about 10% of the total.

The final row in Table 6.2 shows the fractional pressure drop across the various layers of the cornea, calculated from R/R_t, where R is the flow resistance of each individual layer. It is of interest to note that most of the resistance is across the limiting layers (the epithelium and endothelium; Descemet's is too thin to consider here); of the three major layers of the cornea, the stroma, although the thickest layer by far, offers the least resistance to water flow.

PHYSICAL OPTICS

The refractive power of the cornea is easily explained in terms of its curvature and the large difference in refractive index between it and the air. The other optical properties of the cornea, however, those that can be grouped under the heading of "physical optics," are not easily explained. This is especially true for the cornea's most important property: transparency.

Light approaching the corneal surface can be transmitted, reflected, absorbed, scattered, retarded, split (into two rays), or have its plane of polarization altered. Many of these effects have been studied and the influence of species, hydration, and wavelength of light have been reported.

Transmission and Absorption

The most complete recent review of corneal transmission is that of Payrau and co-workers (1967). Figure 6.22 shows the transmission of ultraviolet light (wavelength 210 to 400 nm) through the corneas of several species. As the curves descend, transmission increases. Note that the thresholds for whole corneas of mammals, fish, and birds are all about 280 nm. Figure 6.23 shows an expansion of the upper left-hand cornea of Figure 6.22 and suggests some transmission occurs between 240 and 280 nm for steer and fish corneas. Payrau and associates indicate that the condition of the corneal specimen during measurement, particularly both the time from removal of living eye until measurement and the related extent of drying, may influence the shape of these transmission curves but not the thresholds shown. Data for separate portions of steer cornea, shown in Figures

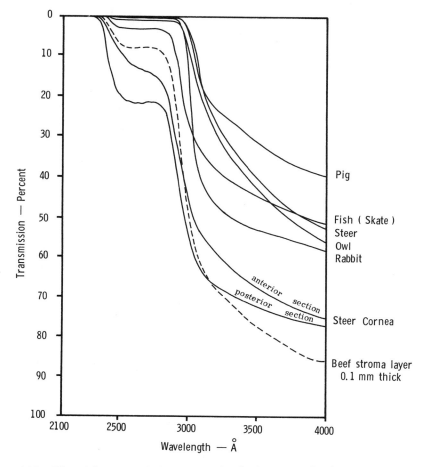

Figure 6.22 Ultraviolet transmission spectra for fresh corneas from several species. (Translated and redrawn from Payrau P, Pouliquen Y, et al. [1967]: La transparence de la cornee. Paris, Masson.)

6.22 and 6.23, suggest that much of the ultraviolet absorption occurs in the corneal epithelium. Figure 6.24 reinforces this conclusion; here transmission for steer epithelium (this sample was three-fourths epithelium and one-fourth stroma as backing) and stroma are shown separately.

Photokeratitis has been known as a primary response of the cornea to ultraviolet absorption for 100 years. Pitts and co-workers (1987) have shown that all layers of the cornea are damaged. Abnormal epithelial cells, damaged and dead keratocytes, and changes in the endothelial cells persist even 8 days after exposure to ultraviolet radiation.

Note also (Figure 6.24) that light transmission through the steer corneal tissues is uniformly greater than 90% above 400 nm. Data for human corneas

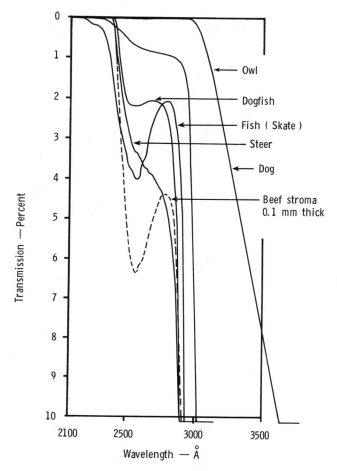

Figure 6.23 Ultraviolet transmission spectra of the cornea for several species. These spectra show details in the range of 0 to 10% transmission. (Translated and redrawn from Payrau P, Pouliquen Y, et al. [1967]: La transparence de la cornee. Paris, Masson.)

were generated by both Lerman (1984) and Beems and Van Best (1990). The latter study suggests that the cornea transmits greater than 90% of incident light for wavelengths greater than about 550 nm and greater than 95% of incident light for wavelengths between 650 and 1000 nm.

Corneal transmission of light in the infrared range, 700 to 3000 nm, varies from species to species and is also dependent on corneal thickness and state of hydration. Figure 6.25 shows that the peaks and valleys of transmission fall at the same wavelengths for shark, owl, and dog corneas, although the transmission rates are different for these animals. The major and distinctive components of the infrared transmission spectrum shown are those of water; the arrows in Figure 6.25 indicate the location of the peaks expected in the transmission spectrum of water.

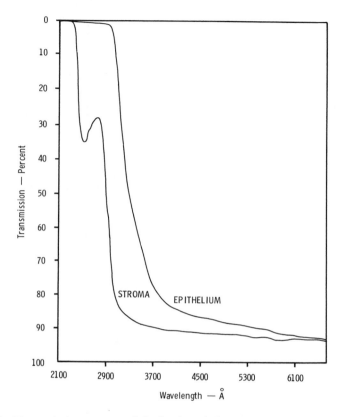

Figure 6.24 Transmission spectra of the beef epithelium and stroma in the ultraviolet and visible wavelengths. (Translated and redrawn from Payrau P, Pouliquen Y, et al. [1967]: La transparence de la cornee. Paris, Masson.)

Early workers immersed corneas in distilled water and observed a gradually increasing loss in transparency; they used the time of immersion rather than corneal hydration as the independent variable. Figure 6.26 demonstrates the effect of immersion time on light transmission through rabbit stroma and whole cornea.

Changes in hydration of the stroma appear to change not only the spectral transmission characteristics but the *shape* of the transmission curve as well. Changes in the transmission profile (for ultraviolet and visible wavelengths) of a section of beef stroma, after up to almost an hour of immersion, are shown in Figure 6.27. Reductions in transmission for light of various specific wavelengths for beef stroma alone (epithelium removed) after various immersion times are shown in Figure 6.28. Figure 6.29 shows similar data, but for just a 0.1-mm thick section of beef cornea stroma, whereas open circles on the same graph indicate the gain in total weight with increased hydration. The curves in Figure 6.30, however, show that immersion of the epithelium alone does not change its transmission characteristics across much of the visible spectrum of light wavelengths.

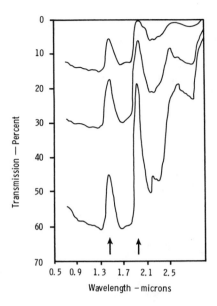

Figure 6.25 Infrared transmission spectra of corneas from three animals. *Top* is dog; *center,* owl; and *bottom,* shark. (Translated and redrawn from Payrau P, Pouliquen Y, et al. [1967]: La transparence de la cornee. Paris, Masson.)

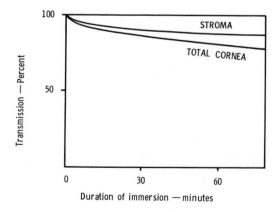

Figure 6.26 Change in light transmission of a rabbit stroma and total cornea as a function of time of immersion in distilled water. (Translated and redrawn from Payrau P, Pouliquen Y, et al. [1967]: La transparence de la cornee. Paris, Masson.)

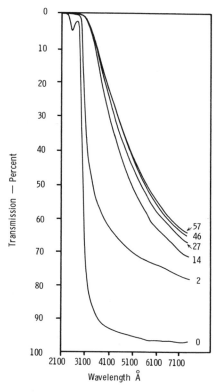

Figure 6.27 Variation in the transmission spectrum in the ultraviolet and visible wavelengths of a beef stroma (0.1 mm thick) when soaked for different times in distilled water. Numbers on the curves indicate the duration of soaking, in minutes. (Translated and redrawn from Payrau P, Pouliquen Y, et al. [1967]: La transparence de la cornee. Paris, Masson.)

Scattering

Although the mammalian cornea is highly transparent in its normal state, transmitting more than 90% of the incident light across a wide band of the visible spectrum, as discussed earlier, an increase in hydration may cause a loss in transparency due to scattering. The nomenclature for studies of scattering in the cornea is shown in Figure 6.31, where a ray of light is shown normally incident to the corneal surface. Figure 6.32 shows scattering as a function of the angle of emergence in rabbit cornea.

Corneal hypoxia from contact lens wear has been associated with both stromal and epithelial edema. It appears that the stroma increases slightly in thickness while the epithelium is stable (O'Leary et al. 1981). Nonetheless, most current research indicates that the visual disturbances (i.e., glare and halos) found with corneal hypoxia secondary specifically to contact lens wear are related more

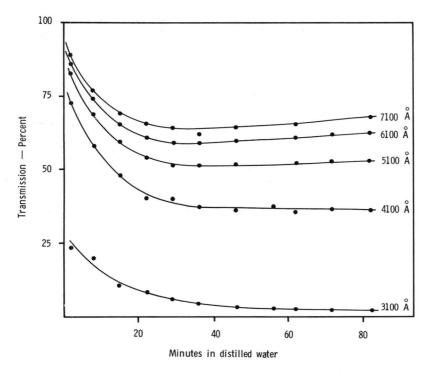

Figure 6.28 Variation in light transmission through a beef cornea denuded of its epithelium as a function of time of immersion in distilled water. Numbers on the curves are wavelength. (Translated and redrawn from Payrau P, Pouliquen Y, et al. [1967]: La transparence de la cornee. Paris, Masson.)

to epithelial scattering and not to stromal changes (Lambert and Klyce 1981; Carney and Jacobs 1984). Epithelial edema, when it occurs, is characterized by large increases in the forward scattering of light and is usually considered more visually disabling than stromal edema (Feuk and McQueen 1971), which induces little scattering until an increase in thickness occurs far greater than that usually seen with contact lens wear. Figure 6.33 shows a direct comparison of scattering and corneal thickness in rabbit cornea. Zucker (1966) monitored his own visual resolution through a rabbit stroma (with epithelium removed) of varying hydration by observing two fine lines whose spacing could be changed. Figure 6.34 shows the angle subtended when two lines could be seen just separately as a function of stromal hydration. In the hydration range of 3 to 6 gm water/gm dry material the two lines could be seen as separate when 2.8 to 3 minutes of arc apart. Above a hydration of 7 gm water/gm dry material the separation had to be greater for the two lines to be distinguishable, and at an extreme of 9 to 10 gm water/gm dry material, visual resolution was only 8 minutes of arc, or only 23% of normal.

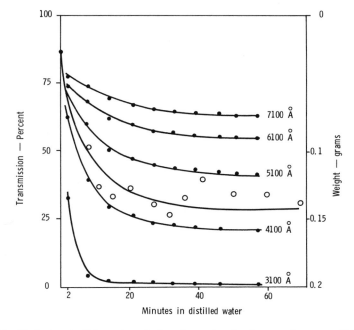

Figure 6.29 Variation in light transmission through a beef corneal stroma (0.1 mm thick) as a function of time of immersion in distilled water. Numbers on the curves are wavelength. Circles show weight increase when read from right-hand axis. (Translated and redrawn from Payrau P, Pouliquen Y, et al. [1967]: La transparence de la cornee. Paris, Masson.)

Care must be taken when considering Zucker's results. Rarely is an *in vivo* human stroma hydrated above 4 to 5 gm water/gm dry weight and yet visual acuity is much lower than would be predicted from Figure 6.34 in these eyes. The clinically observed reduction in visual acuity must therefore be caused by a change in the state of the epithelium, such as discussed earlier with regard to contact lens wear. In fact, visual acuity of an eye with a swollen cornea can be improved 20% to 40% by scraping off the epithelium if this tissue is involved.

Maurice (1957b) has shown that stromal scattering may also occur as a direct result of increased IOP. The curves seen in Figure 6.35 show that scattering increases with increased IOP and thickness (here in percentage of normal thickness, shown by the number on each curve) for rabbit cornea.

Refractive Index

The ratio of the velocity of light in a vacuum to that in any medium is the refractive index of that medium. The refractive index of water, for example, is 1.333—which means that the velocity of light in water is 1/1.33 of that in a

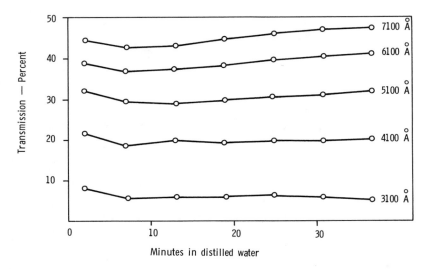

Figure 6.30 Variation of light transmission through the epithelium of the beef cornea as a function of time of immersion in distilled water. Numbers on curves refer to wavelength of incident light. (Translated and redrawn from Payrau P, Pouliquen Y, et al. [1967]: La transparence de la cornee. Paris, Masson.)

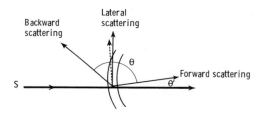

Figure 6.31 Nomenclature for the scattering of light in the cornea. Light is scattered in all directions, but not equally. (Translated and redrawn from Payrau P, Pouliquen Y, et al. [1967]: La transparence de la cornee. Paris, Masson.)

vacuum. The refractive index of human corneal stroma is 1.375 but differs slightly for other species: 1.382 for the ox, and 1.373 for the pig, for examples.

The Gladstone and Dale law of combined refractive index for a composite material can be stated for the corneal stroma as

$$M_s = M_c d_c + M_i d_i \qquad (6.20)$$

where M_s is the refractive index for the stroma, M_c is the refractive index of dry collagen, and M_i that of the ground substance, while d_c and d_i are their volume fractions in the tissue, respectively.

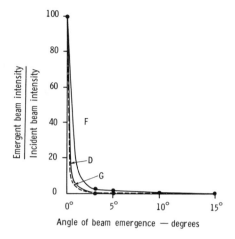

Figure 6.32   Curves showing the scattering of light in the cornea of the rabbit. The ordinate gives the intensity of the light emerging from the cornea, relative to the incident light intensity, as a function of the angle of emergence. (From Kikkawa Y [1960]: Light scattering studies of the rabbit cornea. Jap. J. Physiol. 10:292–302.)

Maurice (1957b) found that $M_c = 1.55$ by immersing pieces of dried stroma in liquids of different refractive indices until a match was found. On the basis that collagen is 60% of the dry weight of the tissue, d_c was estimated at 0.15. M_i was determined by assuming that the ground substance is aqueous humor plus dissolved material:

$$M_i = M_a + \left(\frac{C_s R}{d_i}\right) \tag{6.21}$$

where M_a is the refractive index of aqueous humor (known from independent measurement to be 1.335), C_s is the known concentration of dissolved substances (0.045 gm/ml), and R is the specific refractive index increment, which must lie between 0.19 for proteins and 0.16 for GAG. As $d_i + d_c = 1$, the term d_i is 0.85. An R of 0.18 gives an M_i of 1.345, and from this an M_s of 1.374 is calculated, which is close to the observed value of 1.375, indicating that the stroma follows the Gladstone and Dale law of combined refractive index.

One might expect a large amount of scattering with a two-component system such as described above. Maurice (1957b) calculated that human stroma, with index of collagen fibers at 1.55 and index of the surrounding ground substance at 1.345, should scatter greater than 90% of an incident beam of light at a wavelength of 500 nm. To the contrary, however, the stroma is observed to transmit more than 90% of the incident light. This will be explained below.

Of interest, Fatt and Harris (1973) have shown that the refractive index of the stroma is related to its thickness by the equation

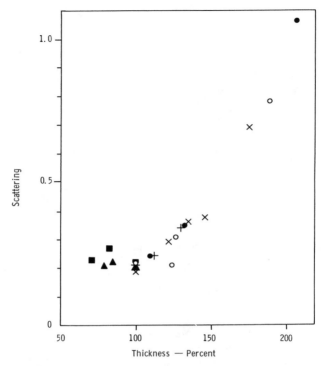

Figure 6.33 Relationship between light back scattered from the cornea and corneal thickness. Green light was shone normally onto the surface of the rabbit cornea and light scattered at 60° to the normal was measured photometrically. The vertical axis gives corneal scattering as the percentage of that which would be obtained if scattering took place from a standard magnesium oxide surface. The horizontal axis shows thickness of the cornea as a percentage of normal. Each symbol represents measurements on one eye for a total of six eyes. Corneas were swollen by placing enucleated eyeball in saline. They were shrunk by replacing aqueous humor by air and leaving at room temperature. (From Maurice DM [1957b]: The structure and transparency of the cornea. J. Physiol. 136:263–286.)

$$M_s = 1.5581 - \left[\frac{(1.89T - 0.189)}{(8.75T - 0.205)}\right] \qquad (6.23)$$

where T is the thickness in milliliters. For human stroma in the normal to clinically observed above-normal range of thicknesses, the refractive index changes, as shown in Figure 6.36. This relationship is useful because it demonstrates that refractive index changes in the cornea during swelling are too small to interfere with its measurement by optical pachometry.

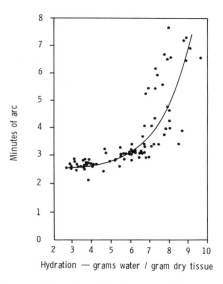

Figure 6.34 Visual acuity as a function of hydration of the stroma. (From Zucker BB [1966]: Arch. Ophthalmol. 75(2):228–231. Copyright 1966. American Medical Association.)

Birefringence

The corneal stroma has two separate indices of refraction for light polarized in different planes. Such an optical system is called *birefringent,* quantitatively stated as simply the difference between the two refractive indices. Maurice (1957b) found a value of 0.00135 for rabbit cornea. Corneal birefringence may be demonstrated by placing a tissue sample between a pair of crossed polarized filters. The birefringence is then indicated by the appearance of a darkened cross pattern on a lighter background; as the tissue is curved, light falling other than at the apex is no longer parallel to the optic axis and a retardation is introduced that produces colored rings seen around the corneal periphery when observing this system.

Birefringence related to the *direction* of the collagen fibrils is called the *textural* birefringence. Alternatively, there is also an *intrinsic* birefringence due to the collagen molecules themselves. The total birefringence observed in the corneal stroma is the sum of the textural and intrinsic birefringences. Maurice (1957b) estimated that the textural birefringence accounts for about 75% of the total. Moreover, the change in observed birefringence when the stroma swells can be predicted from the assumption that all of the incoming water goes into the ground substance (the GAGs). The increased hydration of the GAGs moves the fibrils apart, but the optical properties of the fibrils themselves remain unchanged.

Maurice's study of corneal birefringence led to his description of different indices of refraction for collagen and ground substance, discussed earlier.

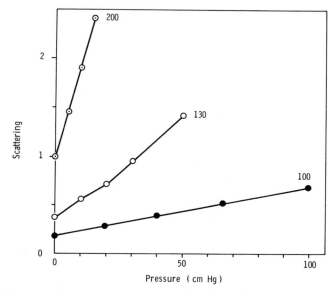

Figure 6.35 Relationship between intraocular pressure and light scattering by the cornea. Pressure in the eye was raised through a needle in the vitreous body. The vertical axis gives corneal scattering as the percentage of that which would be obtained if scattering took place from a standard magnesium oxide surface. The horizontal axis is intraocular pressure. The numbers on the curves represent the thickness of the cornea expressed as a percentage of normal. (From Maurice DM [1957b]: The structure and transparency of the cornea. J. Physiol. 136:263–286.)

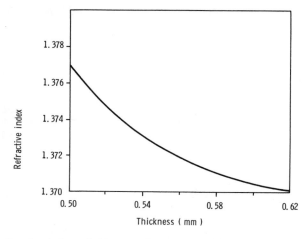

Figure 6.36 Refractive index of the corneal stroma as a function of its thickness. (From Fatt I, Harris MG [1973]: Refractive index of the cornea as a function of its thickness Am. J. Optom. 50:383–386.)

Transparency of the Stroma

A comparison of the cornea with opaque connective tissues like the skin or even the adjacent sclera discloses more similarities than differences. For example, the cornea and sclera share similar collagen fibrils and are about the same in thickness. The cornea, however, acts as a transparent lens, whereas the sclera is sufficiently opaque to form a light-tight chamber for the eye. Maurice (1957b) calculated that a system of collagen fibrils of refractive index 1.55 and 0.10 volume fraction randomly distributed in a ground substance of refractive index 1.345 and 0.90 volume fraction should scatter more than 90% of the incident light; this calculation was discussed earlier and is based on the assumption that each fibril scatters light independently of the other. As the cornea is quite transparent to light in the visible range, this calculation is incorrect, and Maurice became interested in explaining this phenomenon.

Prior to 1957, the explanation for corneal transparency was that the collagen and ground substance had substantially equal refractive indices, but Maurice's study of birefringence in the cornea (also discussed earlier) indicated that this was not so.

Maurice proceeded to make an electron microscope study of the stroma and discovered that the collagen fibrils were not randomly distributed, as he had initially assumed. Instead, the fibrils were found to be arranged in a relatively regular lattice, somewhat like a stack of diffraction gratings. Maurice realized that the transparency of the stroma must be related to the spatial arrangement of the collagen fibrils in a pattern that creates essentially complete destructive interference to light in all directions except forward.

If parallel monochromatic light passes through a grating with its elements separated by a distance *greater* than the wavelength of the light, the scattered radiation is known to recombine only at definite angles to the incident beam. These angles are determined by the ratio of the spacing of the scattering elements to the wavelength of the light; at other angles there is destructive interference. The zero-order image, along the incident beam, is always present and its direction is independent of the spacing of the diffracting elements. As the spacing between the scattering elements decreases, or as the wavelength of the monochromatic light increases, the angles through which the beams of greater than zero order are deviated increases, and fewer images are formed. When the spacing between the scattering elements is equal to the wavelength of incident light, the first-order beam is deviated through 90°. If the spacing is *less* than the wavelength of the light, however, only the zero-order beam remains; the radiation scattered in other directions is suppressed by destructive interference and the grating is transparent.

Therefore, Maurice's theory suggested that stroma is transparent because the axes of its collagen fibrils are arranged in a regular lattice with spacing less than the wavelength of visible light. The spacing in the stroma hypothesized by Maurice is shown in Figure 6.37. Maurice's theory also explained why the stroma becomes cloudy when water is imbibed; more scattering then occurs because the spacing between the collagen fibrils becomes irregular (Figure 6.38) and destructive

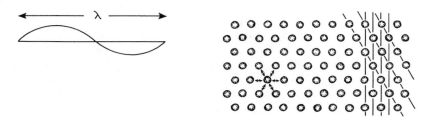

Figure 6.37 Arrangement of fibrils in lattice, shown in section, proposed to explain transparency of cornea. A hexagonal lattice is shown; the lines passing through the fibrils are two sets of lattice planes. The arrows between the fibrils indicate the system of forces that is supposed to maintain the regularity of the structure. The wavelength of light is drawn at the left for comparison. (From Maurice DM [1957]: The structure and transparency of the cornea. J. Physiol. 136:263–286.)

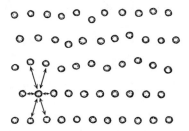

Figure 6.38 Illustration of disorder produced in fibril lattice by swelling. The weakening of the forces of repulsion that keep the row in line is shown schematically. (From Maurice DM [1957]: The structure and transparency of the cornea. J. Physiol. 136:263–286.)

tive interference decreases. Scattering then gives the swollen stroma its milky appearance. Recall Figure 6.33, which shows the increased scattering of the rabbit stroma as it thickens with increased hydration.

The sclera is opaque because, although its fibrils of collagen are parallel over limited regions, their diameters vary greatly (28 to 280 μm), and scleral hydration (2 gm water/gm dry weight) is less than that of the corneal stroma, reflecting a decreased swelling pressure (17 mmHg) and a lower GAG content (about 1%) (Hedbys and Dohlman 1963). The induced light scattering adds to the milky-white appearance of the tissue.

Objections to Maurice's theory came from electron microscopists, who made excellent detailed photographs of the stromal collagen but did not find the *absolute* regularity required by Maurice's theory. Hart and Farrell (1969) then reexamined Maurice's theory and found that the quasiregular and quasirandom spacing and size of the collagen fibrils that they actually observed in the stroma are not inconsistent with transparency according to the Maurice hypothesis. All that

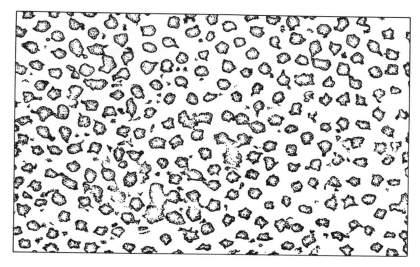

Figure 6.39 Electron micrograph of the rabbit stroma showing the natural spacing of the fibrils. (From Hart RW, Farrell RA [1969]: Light scattering in the cornea. J. Opt. Soc. Am. 59:766.)

is required is that *most* of the spacing be equal. Spacing between the 20- to 30-nm diameter collagen fibers is about 60 nm center to center, leaving spaces of about 30 nm between fibers, and local order extends over distances comparable to the wavelength of visible light. Figure 6.39 shows the natural spacing between the collagen fibrils in an electron micrograph of rabbit stroma. Later, Cox and coworkers (1970) found a marked heterogeneity in the spatial distribution of collagen fibrils in a swollen corneal stroma, consistent with the observed decrease in transparency, further supporting Maurice's theory.

7

Cornea II: Metabolism, Oxygen, Carbon Dioxide, and Contact Lens Wear

The histology of the corneal layers was reviewed at the beginning of chapter 6. Cells in all corneal layers actively metabolize; they must do metabolic work to maintain their temperature, replace cellular components that naturally degrade and decompose, and transport materials across cell membranes. The epithelial cells also metabolize to reproduce.

To perform these metabolic functions, the cells of the cornea require nutrients in the form of glucose, amino acids, and oxygen. Trace amounts of vitamins and minerals are probably also needed. Such materials are delivered to most tissues of the body by the blood of the circulatory system and reach the cells by diffusion from the capillaries without traveling more than a fraction of a millimeter. The cornea, however, is avascular so that (in a teleological sense) it can perform its function of transmitting and refracting light. The nearest blood vessels, in the open eye, are at the limbus—or in the iris and ciliary body. How do nutrients reach the cells of the central cornea that are several millimeters from a blood vessel, and how are metabolic waste products removed?

It was once believed that the blood vessels of the limbus were the direct source of corneal nutrients. Many experiments have now been performed to demonstrate that the limbal vessels play a minor role, if any, in the nutrition of the cornea. If a deep cut is made completely around the periphery of the cornea, for example, there appears to be no impairment of central corneal physiology. Maurice (1967) provided additional support for this argument: he ingested fluorescein so that a constant concentration level of the dye was maintained in his own blood for 12 hours. The concentration of dye in his cornea and aqueous humor was measured at the end of this period. His results show that most material diffusing inward from the limbus into the cornea will be lost from the cornea by passage through either of the two surfaces and little if any finally diffuses through to the central zone. It must be concluded that the potential sources of *in vivo* corneal nutrition of the open eye are the aqueous humor and tears. It is believed that the tears offer only oxygen, whereas some oxygen and all the glucose, amino acids, and other nutrients must come from the aqueous humor. In the instance of the closed eye (during sleep), the capillaries of the palpebral conjunctiva become a source of corneal nutrition and may carry off waste products.

It must be emphasized that the transport of nutrients and waste products through the cornea is by diffusion and not through convective or bulk flow of the water phase in the cornea (see Chapter 6 for descriptions of these processes). Bert and Fatt (1969) have shown that the diffusion process is predominant because of the very low velocity of liquid flow in the cornea.

GLUCOSE

The metabolic reaction of oxygen and glucose that provides energy for the various cellular functions is called *respiration*. Energy in the form of adenosine triphosphate (ATP) is generated by the breakdown of 1 mole of glucose to water and carbon dioxide, first by the Embden-Meyerhof pathway (*anaerobic glycolysis*) yielding 2 moles of ATP. In the absence of oxygen, this process ends here in pyruvic acid, which is then converted to lactic acid. If oxygen is available, the conventional tricarboxylic acid (TCA) or Kreb cycle (*aerobic glycolysis*) usually follows, taking pyruvic acid to CO_2 and water to yield an additional 36 moles of ATP. Kinoshita and colleagues (1955) estimated that 65% of the glucose utilized by *in vitro* bovine corneas exposed to 95% oxygen was oxidized by the TCA cycle, and 35% was oxidized by way of an alternative hexose monophosphate shunt. The TCA cycle may not be very active in the *in vivo* epithelium, however, as it is located in mitochondria, which are sparse, especially in the superficial layers. Riley (1969) determined that only about 15% of rabbit corneal glucose is fully oxidized under normal conditions; the bulk is anaerobically converted to lactic acid as an end product. As we have discussed, production of lactic acid is usually an indication that cells are receiving insufficient oxygen for complete oxidation of glucose. The cornea, however, as discussed earlier, is a thin tissue with its cellular boundary layers in intimate contact with oxygen-containing fluids on both sides; the high rate of lactic acid production therefore remains an unexplained observation in corneal physiology. The disposal of lactic acid will be seen to be quite important. Detailed descriptions of these biochemical reactions are beyond the scope of this text. The interested reader is referred to the discussion by Maurice and Riley (1968).

The tear film might be intuitively accepted as a potential major source of glucose for the epithelium because of its proximity. Epithelial permeability to glucose, however, as with other water-soluble compounds, is low. Tears also have a very low glucose concentration (only about 3 mg/100 ml according to Dohlman [1971]) and probably cannot supply corneal needs, found to be about 100 μg/cm^2 hour in the rabbit (Riley, 1969). The epithelium alone probably consumes 20 μg/cm^2 hour or more (Thoft and Friend 1971).

The source of glucose for respiration in the cells of the cornea is therefore believed to be the aqueous humor, where the concentration is 124 mg/100 ml, or 40 times that of the tears. Dohlman (1971) reported that experiments with intrastromal membranes, or with silicone oil in the anterior chamber, support this view. Both glucose and glycogen drastically decrease in the anterior tissues after imposing these barriers, and corneal degeneration may follow. Hale and Maurice (1969) found that both glucose and methyl glucose enter the cornea at rates double those expected from simple diffusion. They postulated a facilitated process for moving glucose from the aqueous humor across the endothelium into the stroma.

The steady-state glucose concentration in the epithelium is about 70 mg/100 gm wet weight. As the biological half-life of glucose in cells is about 8 minutes at 37°C, corneal glucose should be almost completely exhausted in about 16 minutes if the external re-supply is eliminated. One might note that at 27°C this glucose will last 32 minutes and at 17°C 64 minutes. Another potential source of metabolic energy, however, is stored glycogen (primarily in the epithelium), which amounts to about 2 mg/gm of whole cornea. If there is an interruption in external glucose supply, after the glucose dissolved in the cornea is exhausted, the cornea will use its stored glycogen at the rate of 50 μg/hour per gram of whole cornea until this supply is also totally consumed.

It will be useful in subsequent discussion of corneal physiology to consider the energy released by biochemical oxidation of glucose in the cornea. Maurice (1969) estimated that oxidation in the endothelium should release about 10^{-3} cal/cm^2 hour. No quantitative data are available for the other layers of the cornea. As the stroma develops an imbibition pressure that would cause swelling, work must be done against this pressure to keep the cornea at a constant thickness. The energy requirment of such a process was calculated to be about 8×10^{-6} cal/cm^2 hour. We conclude from these data that sufficient energy is available to maintain normal corneal thickness in the face of the ever-present imbibition pressure.

Complete oxidation of glucose yields carbon dioxide and water. Disposal of carbon dioxide will be discussed below together with the analysis of oxygen movement in the cornea since both are dissolved gases. The respiratory quotient of the ox cornea was found to be 1.00 by de Roetth (1950), so the amount of oxygen consumed is equal to the amount of carbon dioxide produced. We noted above that about 80% of the glucose, however, is incompletely oxidized to lactic acid, and this must also be removed from the tissue.

AMINO ACIDS

The constant shedding and replacement by mitosis of the epithelial cells require a continuous supply of amino acids to allow synthesis of proteins. It appears that amino acids are also supplied from the aqueous humor, principally by passive diffusion. Cell membrane permeability values for amino acids are close to those predicted on the basis of their molecular sizes (see Chapter 6). Amino acids in quantities sufficient to permit the synthesis of some 10 μg/hour of protein by the epithelial cells can enter by diffusion, but an additional influx by facilitated transport has not been totally ruled out (Riley 1977).

OXYGEN

The movement of oxygen in the cornea is important when analyzing the effects of contact lens wear. One should note, however, that even in the absence of a contact lens the state of hydration and health of the cornea seem intimately connected with the availability of oxygen to this tissue.

Corneal Oxygen Requirements (Without a Contact Lens)

It was long suspected that the avascular cornea derived all or part of the oxygen needed for its cellular respiration directly from the air (Smelser and Ozanics 1952). The first quantitative report of this consumption was made by Hill and Fatt (1963b), who used a Clark-type polarographic oxygen sensor to monitor the depletion of oxygen by human corneas from an air-saturated solution in a small chamber that was built into a scleral contact lens (Figure 7.1). A membrane separates this sensor's cathode and anode from the sample being tested. The potential between the cathode and anode is maintained at about 0.7 volt, and

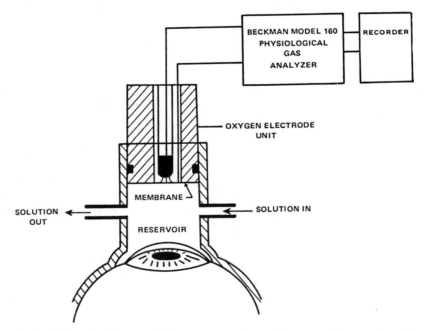

Figure 7.1 Schematic diagram of the oxygen sensor and lens assemblies used to obtain data for calculating the rate of oxygen consumption by the cornea *in vivo*. (From Hill RM, Fatt I [1964]: Oxygen measurements under a contact lens. Am. J. Optom. 41:382–387.)

under these conditions oxygen is the only species expected to accept electrons. Current, therefore, is directly related to the diffusion of oxygen molecules across the membrane into the space between the anode and cathode within the sensor. This current is proportional to the concentration of oxygen at the outer surface of the membrane.

The time course of oxygen tension change found in the chamber with this device on a human eye is shown in Figure 7.2; oxygen flux into the cornea was calculated from this figure to be about 4.8 μl O_2/cm^2 hour. Oxygen uptake was found to decrease as the oxygen tension in the reservoir decreased. Haberich (1966) sampled the volumetric concentration of oxygen over time in a gas-filled chamber (covering a freshly enucleated bovine eye) by a modified Krogh microgas analysis device (Figure 7.3) and found this same effect. Data from both of these studies are summarized in Table 7.1.

Neither of these methods is clinically useful. Both methods are too slow and require great technical skill. Furthermore, because they are slow, large numbers of measurements cannot be made in a reasonable time. For this reason, Hill and Fatt (1963a) simplified their earlier procedure by replacing the scleral contact lens device with a sensor covered by a thin polyethylene membrane; in this method the oxygen reservoir is the membrane itself (Figure 7.4). Because the membrane is so thin (12 to 20 μm), the oxygen supply is very small and is therefore depleted very

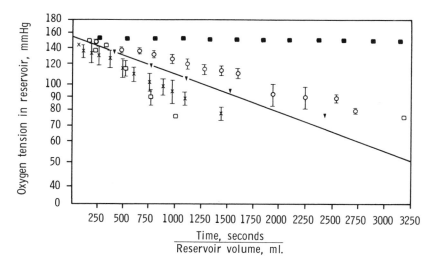

Figure 7.2 Oxygen tension in the reservoir shown as a function of the parameter time divided by reservoir volume. *x*, for 0.83 μl, reservoir volume; ○, for 0.62 μl; □, for 0.20 μl, using the sensor shown in Figure 7.1. Vertical lines represent one standard deviation about the mean of several determinations at each reservoir volume. The solid line is the best estimate regression line. ■, the response of the electrode assembly when pressed against a surface impermeable to oxygen. (From Hill RM, Fatt I [1963]: J. Am. Optom. Assoc. 142:1295–1297. Copyright 1963 by the American Association for the Advancement of Science.)

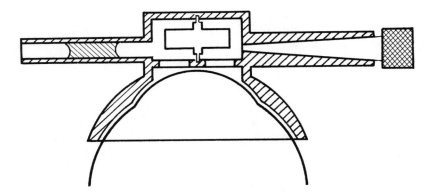

Figure 7.3 Haberich's volumetric method for measuring the oxygen uptake of the cornea. (From Haberich FJ [1966]: Quelques aspects physiologiques de l'adaption des verres de contact. Cahiers Verres Cont. 11:1–6.)

Table 7.1 Oxygen Flux (j) into the Cornea (in $\mu l/cm^2$ hour)

Oxygen Tension (in mmHg)	Hill and Fatt (1963b) (Human Data)	Haberich (1966) (Bovine Data)
155	4.8	9.0
100	3.1	8.0
50	1.5	6.0

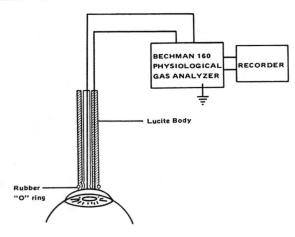

Figure 7.4 Schematic drawing of an oxygen sensor being applied to a cornea. The rubber "O" ring holds a polyethylene membrane on the end of the sensor. The cornea removes the oxygen from this membrane to give the record shown by ■ in Figure 7.5. (From Fatt I [1976]: The polarographic oxygen sensor. CRC Press Inc. Reprinted with permission of CRC Press Inc.)

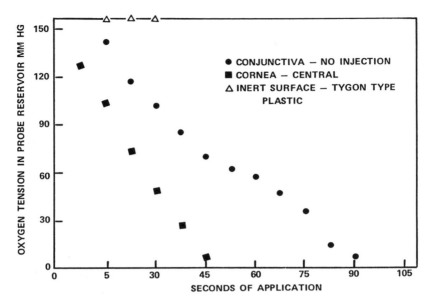

Figure 7.5   Graphical representation of fall in oxygen tension in sensor membrane when the probe is pressed against three different surfaces. (From Hill RM, Fatt I [1964]: Oxygen measurements under a contact lens. Am. J. Optom. 41:382–387. Reprinted with permission of the *Journal of the American Optometric Association.*)

rapidly. When this membrane-covered sensor is held against a cornea, oxygen is depleted in 1 to 2 minutes (Figure 7.5). This procedure, however, although rapid, is not very accurate. It is also worth noting that both Farris and co-workers (1965) and Jauregui and Fatt (1972) suggest that such rapid depletion means that these data represent primarily *epithelial* oxygen consumption.

Because of the lack of accuracy, this method has been primarily used to compare *relative oxygen flux rates*. It is useful when the effect of a drug or a contact lens on oxygen uptake is under study. The measured oxygen uptake may then be compared to that found with a control eye that has not been treated or covered with a contact lens. The corneal response found with one contact lens in place might be compared with that from a different contact lens, for another example.

When the membrane-covered sensor is pressed against the cornea, the oxygen tension inside the sensor decreases, as is shown in Figure 7.5. Hill and Fatt (1964) used the time for a drop in recorded oxygen tension from 140 mmHg to 100 mmHg as the rate of oxygen uptake by the cornea, but this procedure is quite arbitrary as the relationship between oxygen tension and time is clearly not linear. Farris and colleagues (1965) suggested ignoring the early drop in oxygen tension because it is too "noisy," but this is also arbitrary. Jauregui and Fatt (1971) presented another method to convert these data to quantitative numbers.

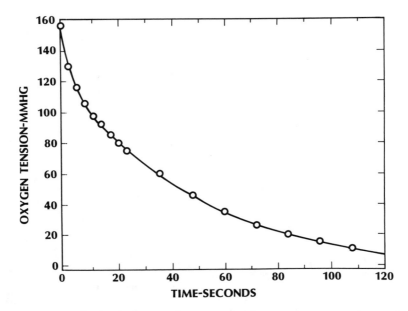

Figure 7.6 A typical record on an arithmetic scale of oxygen tension in the membrane of the sensor shown in Figure 7.4. The sensor was placed on the cornea at time zero after having been previously exposed to air in which the oxygen content is 20% and the oxygen tension is 155 mmHg. (From Weissman BA [1979]: Reversal of the effects of corneal anoxia by oxygen breathing. PhD thesis, University of California, Berkeley.)

Inspection of such a record (Figure 7.6) suggests that the drop in oxygen tension may be exponential with time. Data are plotted on a semilog graph in Figure 7.7, and the straight-line fit can be described by the equation

$$\frac{d\log P}{dt} = a \text{ constant}_1 \tag{7.1}$$

where P is the oxygen tension and t is time. In natural logarithms

$$\frac{d\log_e P}{dt} = a \text{ constant}_2 \tag{7.2}$$

From the calculus we have

$$\frac{d\log_e P}{dt} = \frac{(dP)}{(Pdt)} \tag{7.3}$$

The fall in oxygen tension inside the membrane must be a result of oxygen leaving the membrane and going into the cornea; this rate can be written as

$$\frac{dP}{dt} = \frac{j}{Lk} \tag{7.4}$$

where j is the rate of oxygen uptake by the cornea in milliliters per square centimeter per second (ml/cm^2 sec), L is the membrane thickness in centimeters, and k is the solubility of oxygen in the membrane (from Henry's law) given as

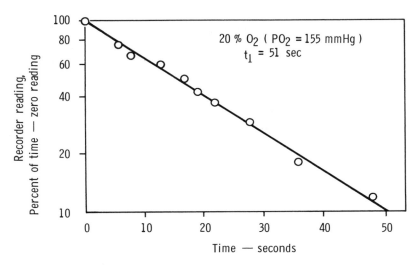

Figure 7.7 A typical record on a semilogarithmic scale of oxygen tension in the membrane of the sensor shown in Figure 7.4. The sensor was placed on the cornea at time zero after having been previously exposed to air in which oxygen content is 20% and oxygen tension is 155 mmHg. The ordinate is a logarithmic scale that takes 100% as the reading at time zero. The straight line falls by a factor of 10 on the ordinate scale in 51 seconds.

milliliters of oxygen per milliliter per millimeter of mercury (ml O_2/ml mmHg). Substituting the term for dP/dt from Equation 7.4 into Equation 7.3

$$\frac{d\log_e P}{dt} = \frac{j}{PLk} \tag{7.5}$$

and rearrangement gives

$$j = PkL \left(\frac{d\log_e P}{dt}\right) \tag{7.6}$$

When P falls by a factor of 10, $d\log_e P$ is 2.3 and the time for this to happen is t_1. Equation 7.6 becomes

$$j = 2.3 \frac{PLk}{t_1} \tag{7.7}$$

and j is therefore the corneal oxygen uptake rate found at the oxygen tension P. Jauregui and Fatt (1972) measured the corneal oxygen uptake of a human subject exposed to air ($P = 155$ mmHg) and found a value of about 3 μl O_2/cm² hour; as noted above, they suggested that this rate represents primarily epithelial consumption. Larke and co-workers (1981) used a version of this method on a series of 68 male Caucasian subjects (ranging in age from 18 to 25 years) and found a distribution in oxygen uptake rate ranging from 3 to 9 μl O_2/cm² hour, with the mean at 6 μl O_2/cm² hour.

160 | PHYSIOLOGY OF THE EYE

The Critical Oxygen Tension

Another approach to the study of corneal oxygen consumption is by means
of the so-called critical oxygen tension or COT. Using a goggle through which
humidified gases of known oxygen concentrations were passed, Polse and Mandell (1971) were the first to suggest that there was a COT value below which the
cornea would receive insufficient oxygen to maintain its thickness (the mechanism
of this change is both interesting and important and will be discussed in detail
later). They found that human corneal swelling occurred when the oxygen tension
over the anterior corneal surface fell below 11 to 19 mmHg. The oxygen tension
of room air is normally 21% of the barometric pressure (760 mmHg at sea level),
or about 155 mmHg. The middle of the range 11 to 19 mmHg is 15 mmHg.
Mandell and Farrell (1980) subsequently increased this value to 23 to 35 mmHg,
and Holden and colleagues (1984) increased it again to about 70 mmHg. In
both larger and more controlled goggle studies (Figure 7.8), it should be re-
membered that Holden and co-workers' COT of 70 mmHg is above that of the
oxygen tension in the palpebral conjunctiva. Since the cornea is covered with
the palpebral conjunctiva during the one-third of our lives spent sleeping, it is
difficult to accept a COT that is higher than the normal palpebral conjunctival
oxygen tension.

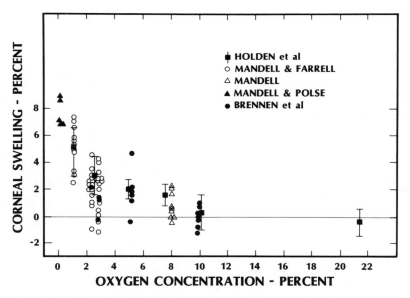

Figure 7.8 Relationship between oxygen concentration, stated as volume percent in gas
at the precorneal surface, and corneal swelling after 3 hours. (From Mandell RB
[1988]: Contact Lens Practice, 4th ed. Springfield, IL, Charles C Thomas. With
permission.)

Others have looked at alternative corneal functions to define the minimal anterior corneal oxygen tension that will not induce metabolic compromise. Uniacke and associates (1972) found that an oxygen tension of 40 mmHg (5% oxygen) was needed to prevent glycogen depletion in the rabbit epithelium. Millidot and O'Leary (1980) found that human corneal touch sensitivity decreased if anterior corneal oxygen tension fell below about 60 mmHg. Hamano and coworkers (1983) found changes in lactate production and epithelial mitosis rate in the rabbit if the anterior corneal oxygen tension was below 100 mmHg, and Masters (1984) found changes in the rabbit mitochondria redox state when anterior corneal oxygen tension was below about 75 mmHg. Again, it is difficult to understand reports of abnormal corneal cell behavior at oxygen tensions above that of the normal palpebral conjunctiva.

Freeman (1972) measured *in vitro* oxygen consumption rates for separate layers of excised rabbit cornea: epithelium, stroma, and endothelium. A polarographic procedure, not unlike that of Hill and Fatt (1963a) or Jauregui and Fatt (1971), was used. Freeman's data are shown in the first and second columns of Table 7.2; both columns display the oxygen consumption rate but different units are used. The last column shows the permeability term $(D_e k)$ found for diffusion of oxygen in the separate layers; these data are from Freeman and Fatt (1972). Weissman and associates (1983) later found a value similar to that of Freeman and Fatt (1972) for the $D_e k$ of oxygen in human stroma: 29.5×10^{-11} ml O_2 cm^2/ml mmHg sec.

Oxygen Flux and Distribution of Oxygen in the Cornea

Table 7.2 gives the data needed to calculate the flux of dissolved oxygen diffusing across each layer of the cornea. Equation 6.4 from the preceding chapter is restated and will be used to make these calculations with v (the volume of dissolved oxygen in milliliters at STP) substituted for m for simplicity:

Table 7.2 Oxygen Consumption Rate (Q) and Oxygen Permeability $(D_e k)$ of Excised Rabbit Cornea at 37° C*

Layer	Q *(ml O_2/ml sec)*	Q'† *(μl O_2/cm^2 hour)*	$D_e k$ *(ml cm^2 ml mmHg sec)*
Epithelium	26.5×10^{-5}	3.83	12.2×10^{-11}
Stroma	2.85×10^{-5}	3.68	30.0×10^{-11}
Endothelium	140.0×10^{-5}	2.03	2.7×10^{-11}
Whole cornea	6.58×10^{-5}	9.54	24.7×10^{-11}

*Data from Freeman RD (1972): Oxygen consumption by the component layers of the cornea. J. Physiol. 225:15–32; and Freeman and Fatt (1972)

†Q' is the amount of oxygen that passes into a square centimeter of tissue per hour. It is calculated from the Q values shown and the thicknesses given in Table 6.2.

$$J = \frac{dv}{dt} = -\frac{D_e\, a\, \Delta C}{L} \tag{7.8}$$

Recall that the minus sign here indicates diffusion is down a concentration gradient. Since it is more convenient to speak of flux, which is rate per unit area, we again define j as the flux and equal to J/a. Then

$$j = -\frac{D_e\, \Delta C}{L} \tag{7.9}$$

We will start with a single-layer model cornea where elementary calculus can be used to obtain a set of equations to predict both oxygen flux into the cornea and the steady-state distribution of oxygen within the tissue.

The cornea is thin compared to its area, so all oxygen movement may be considered to occur normal to the surface. We then have a one-dimensional problem, as shown in Figure 7.9. An element of tissue with thickness of L along the x direction has been chosen in which there is oxygen movement into and out of the material. Equation 7.9 tells us that the oxygen flux *into* this element at position x will be

$$j_{\text{in at } x} = -D_e \left(\frac{dC}{dx}\right)_x \tag{7.10}$$

At another position, $x + dx$, similarly, the flux *out* of this element is

$$J_{\text{out at } x+dx} = -D_e \left(\frac{dC}{dx}\right)_{x+dx} \tag{7.11}$$

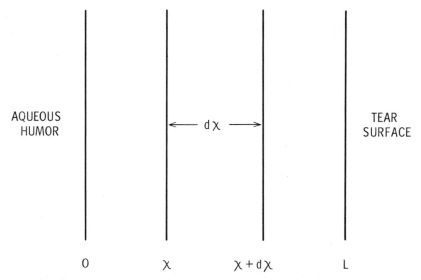

Figure 7.9 Model of a cornea treated as a one-dimensional single layer.

If we subtract Equation 7.11 from 7.10 and simplify, we obtain an expression for the difference in flux as oxygen diffuses across the element of thickness dx. Stated mathematically this is

$$j_x - j_{x+dx} = -D_e \left[\left(\frac{dC}{dx}\right)_{x+dx} - \left(\frac{dC}{dx}\right)_x \right] \qquad (7.12)$$

The left-hand side of Equation 7.12 says there has been a change of flux across the element of thickness dx. The change in flux can be written as $j_x - j_{x+dx} = dj$. Therefore

$$\frac{j_x - j_{x+dx}}{dx} = \frac{dj}{dx} \qquad (7.13)$$

The right-hand side of Equation 7.12 says there has been a change in dC/dx, and this can be written as

$$\frac{(dC/dx)_{x+dx} - (dC/dx)_x}{dx} = \frac{[d(dC/dx)]}{dx} \qquad (7.14)$$

Substituting the results of Equations 7.13 and 7.14 back into Equation 7.12

$$\frac{dj}{dx} = -D_e \left[\frac{d(dC/dx)}{dx} \right] \qquad (7.15)$$

Carrying out the differentiation indicated on the right-hand side of Equation 7.15 gives

$$\frac{dj}{dx} = -\frac{D_e \, d^2 C}{dx^2} \qquad (7.16)$$

Since we are considering a steady-state situation, the only way there can be a change in flux dj/dx across dx is if oxygen is consumed or produced in the element dx. There are no sources of oxygen production in the cornea. We will call the consumption rate Q. The reader should note that consumption of the diffusing species is indicated by a positive value of Q here, and that production—of carbon dioxide, for example—would require use of a negative value for Q. The amount of oxygen consumed within the element must be equal to Q multiplied by a volume that is the area times the thickness, or QaL. Therefore, the total change in volume of oxygen over time in this element is equal to the change in flux times the area plus the consumption, or

$$\frac{dv}{dt} = \Delta ja + QaL \qquad (7.17)$$

As v also equals the concentration of dissolved gas times volume of solution or tissue, or CaL, this means that

$$aL \left[\frac{dC}{dt} \right] = \Delta ja + QaL \qquad (7.18)$$

and dividing both sides by aL (where $L = \Delta x$)

$$\frac{dC}{dt} = \frac{dj}{dx} + Q \tag{7.19}$$

Substituting for dj/dx from Equation 7.16

$$\frac{dC}{dt} = \left[-\frac{D_e\, d^2C}{dx^2}\right] + Q \tag{7.20}$$

Now, from Henry's law, $C = kP$, so Equation 7.20 becomes

$$k\left[\frac{dP}{dt}\right] = \left[-\frac{D_e k\, d^2P}{dx^2}\right] + Q \tag{7.21}$$

but in the steady state $dP/dt = 0$, so Equation 7.21 becomes

$$\left[-\frac{D_e k\, d^2P}{dx^2}\right] + Q = 0 \tag{7.22}$$

which becomes, with division by $-D_e k$

$$\frac{d^2P}{dx^2} - \left[\frac{Q}{D_e k}\right] = 0 \tag{7.23}$$

or $d^2P/dx^2 = Q/D_e k$. This indicates that the second derivative of P with respect to x is a constant $(Q/D_e k)$, and from the calculus we know that the first derivative must have been

$$\frac{dP}{dx} = \left[\frac{Qx}{D_e k}\right] + B \tag{7.24}$$

where B is a constant whose value we will have to determine later when we set the boundary conditions. We can rearrange Equation 7.24 to

$$dP = \left[\frac{Qx}{D_e k}\right]dx + B\,dx \tag{7.25}$$

and integration of Equation 7.25 then gives

$$P = \left[\frac{Qx^2}{2D_e k}\right] + [Bx] + C \tag{7.26}$$

C is a constant of integration and is the sum of constants of integration of all three integrations in Equation 7.25. Equation 7.26 is the *general solution* of Equation 7.23 because we have not yet specified the conditions that will give values of the integration constants B and C.

Four conditions may now be applied to this mathematical model of the cornea. In all cases the posterior cornea is in contact with the aqueous humor. It has already been stated (see Chapter 2) that direct measurements of oxygen tension in the aqueous humor of the air-breathing rabbit led to values ranging from 25 to 75 mmHg; we shall therefore use 55 mmHg as the best estimate for oxygen tension of the posterior corneal boundary.

The four cases are:

1. The open eye, where the anterior surface of the cornea is covered by a film of air-saturated tears.
2. The closed eye, where the anterior surface is covered by the palpebral conjunctiva.
3. The eye in an oxygen-free environment; this is the case of the nitrogen goggle experiment, discussed earlier, in its extreme; the anterior corneal surface is open to an atmosphere that contains nitrogen and perhaps water vapor, but no oxygen.
4. The covered eye, where the anterior surface is covered with a contact lens. Several subdivisions of this condition are of interest: there is the rigid lens that may allow tear exchange, and the hydrogel lens that does not, and both can be present on the eye under open or closed eyelid conditions, and both can have varying oxygen transmissibility values (including zero).

The Open Eye

We assume that the tears over the cornea of the open eye are saturated with air. This means that the boundary layer oxygen tension is 155 mmHg (at sea level). Adopting the coordinate system shown in Figure 7.9 we can now write our boundary conditions as

$$x = 0, P = 55 \text{ mmHg}$$
$$x = L, P = 155 \text{ mmHg} \tag{7.27}$$

where L is the thickness of the cornea. It is now a simple matter to evaluate B and C in Equation 7.26. If $P = 55$ mmHg for $x = 0$, then C must be 55 mmHg. Setting $C = 55$ mmHg and $P = 155$ mmHg for $x = L$, B will be found by substituting these values into Equation 7.26:

$$155 \text{ mmHg} = \left[\frac{QL^2}{2D_ek}\right] + BL + 55 \text{ mmHg} \tag{7.28}$$

and then rearrangement gives

$$B = \left[\frac{1}{L}\right] \left(100 \text{ mmHg} - \left[\frac{QL^2}{2D_ek}\right]\right) \tag{7.29}$$

The equation that gives P as a function of x for the open eye is now obtained by substituting the above results for B and C back into Equation 7.26:

$$P = \left[\frac{Qx^2}{2D_ek}\right] + \left(\frac{x}{L}\right) \left(100 \text{ mmHg} - \left[\frac{QL^2}{2D_ek}\right]\right) + 55 \text{ mmHg} \tag{7.30}$$

If Q/D_ek and L are known for the cornea, we can substitute these values, together with a set of x values, into Equation 7.30 and determine the oxygen tension at each point across the cornea.

We must digress here for a moment to discuss what Equation 7.30 tells us about the oxygen flux into the cornea. Recall from Equation 6.5 that flux, symbolized by j, is the amount of oxygen that crosses any surface per unit surface area per unit time. Using Henry's law to convert concentration to oxygen tension we have

$$j = -D_e k \left[\frac{dP}{dx}\right] \tag{7.31}$$

The term dP/dx can be obtained by differentiating Equation 7.30 to give

$$\frac{dP}{dx} = \left[\frac{Qx}{D_e k}\right] + \left(\frac{1}{L}\right)(100 \text{ mmHg} - \left[\frac{QL^2}{2D_e k}\right]) \tag{7.32}$$

If we wish to determine the flux at the posterior surface of the cornea, for example, where $x = 0$, we start by setting x to 0 in Equation 7.32 to give

$$\left(\frac{dP}{dx}\right)_{x=0} = \left(\frac{1}{L}\right)(100 \text{ mmHg} - \left[\frac{QL^2}{2D_e k}\right]) \tag{7.33}$$

Substituting this result into Equation 7.31, we obtain

$$j_{x=0} = -D_e k \left(\frac{1}{L}\right)(100 \text{ mmHg} - \left[\frac{QL^2}{2D_e k}\right]) \tag{7.34}$$

or, simplifying

$$j_{x=0} = \left(\frac{QL}{2}\right) - \left(100 \text{ mmHg} \frac{D_e k}{L}\right) \tag{7.35}$$

To find the flux at the anterior surface of the cornea, where $x = L$, we make this substitution in Equation 7.32 to find

$$\left(\frac{dP}{dx}\right)_{x=L} = \left(\frac{QL}{D_e k}\right) + \left(\frac{1}{L}\right)\left(100 \text{ mmHg} - \left[\frac{QL^2}{2D_e k}\right]\right) \tag{7.36}$$

which simplifies to

$$\left(\frac{dP}{dx}\right)_{x=L} = \left(\frac{QL}{2D_e k}\right) + \left(\frac{100 \text{ mmHg}}{L}\right) \tag{7.37}$$

Substituting Equation 7.37 into Equation 7.31

$$j_{x=L} = -\left(\left[\frac{QL}{2}\right] + \left[100 \text{ mmHg} \frac{D_e k}{L}\right]\right) \tag{7.38}$$

If we compare Equations 7.35 and 7.38 we see that Equation 7.35 predicts a flux in the left-to-right direction (see Figure 7.9) with a magnitude of $QL/2$ minus a diffusion term 100 mmHg $D_e k/L$. On the other hand, Equation 7.38 predicts a flux in the right-to-left direction with a magnitude of $QL/2$ plus the diffusion term 100 mmHg $D_e k/L$. Furthermore, the total flux j into the cornea without regard to direction is QL. This is exactly as we could have predicted because the units of flux are ml $O_2/cm^2 \times$ sec whereas consumption Q is ml $O_2/ml \times$ sec. As L is in centimeters, QL is in milliliters of $O_2/cm^2 \times$ sec or j.

Although the total flux into the cornea is QL, this total is not equally divided between the anterior and posterior surfaces for the boundary conditions of Equation 7.27. A comparison of Equations 7.35 and 7.38 shows that there is a greater flux, by an amount of 200 mmHg $D_e k/L$, coming into the anterior than into posterior surface.

The Closed Eye

The case of the closed eye is only a little different from that of the open eye. Oxygen tension in the aqueous remains at 55 mmHg, or $P = 55$ mmHg at $x = 0$. The anterior surface of the cornea of the closed eye is covered by the palpebral conjunctiva. Fatt and Bieber (1968), Kwan and Fatt (1970), Efron and Carney (1979), and Isenberg and Green (1985) all indicate the oxygen tension of this surface should be about 55 mmHg as well. We can therefore take $P = 55$ mmHg at $x = L$. These two conditions are now used to evaluate B and C in Equation 7.26. As above, $C = 55$ mmHg, and then

$$B = -\left[\frac{QL}{2D_e k}\right] \tag{7.39}$$

The equation for P as a function of x now becomes

$$P = \left[\frac{Qx^2}{2D_e k}\right] - \left[\frac{QLx}{2D_e k}\right] + 55 \text{ mmHg} \tag{7.40}$$

The calculation of flux into the anterior and posterior surfaces of the cornea of the closed eye proceeds in the same way as for the open eye. In the case of the closed eye, however, because P is set at 55 mmHg at both surfaces, the flux at each surface is exactly $QL/2$.

The Cornea in an Oxygen-Free Environment

Oxygen tension is zero at the anterior corneal surface under the conditions of a nitrogen goggle experiment; oxygen is excluded by passing humidified nitrogen over the anterior surface of the cornea (Polse and Mandell 1970). Carbon dioxide or other gases could be used here as well but might change the physiological results in certain ways. The differential equation whose solution will give corneal oxygen tension as a function of position is still 7.23, and the general solution still applicable is Equation 7.26.

We can again set $P = 55$ mmHg at $x = 0$ for the aqueous humor at the posterior corneal surface. Some believe that conditions on the anterior corneal surface influence oxygen tension in the aqueous humor (Barr and Silver 1973), but this experimental evidence is flimsy and has been challenged (Weissman et al. 1981). From Equation 7.26 this condition again gives $C = 55$ mmHg.

At the boundary $x = L$, we let $P = 0$, to agree with the conditions of the nitrogen goggle. Using Equation 7.26 and solving for B

$$B = -\left[\frac{QL}{2D_ek}\right] - \left[\frac{55 \text{ mmHg}}{L}\right] \qquad (7.41)$$

Substituting these results for B and C into Equation 7.26 gives the relationship of oxygen tension to position in our one-layer model cornea:

$$P = \left[\frac{Qx^2}{2D_ek}\right] - \left(\left[\frac{QL}{2D_ek}\right] + \left[\frac{55 \text{ mmHg}}{L}\right]\right)x + 55 \text{ mmHg} \qquad (7.42)$$

We will return to the discussion of the physical meaning of Equation 7.42 in the real world after we examine a similar case in which oxygen supply to the anterior corneal surface is blocked by a tight-fitting oxygen-impermeable contact lens.

The Tight Oxygen-Impermeable Contact Lens

Again $P = 55$ mmHg at $x = 0$, and therefore $C = 55$ mmHg. But at $x = L$, the tight oxygen-impermeable contact lens means that $j = 0$ at this boundary. We know that $j = -D_ek\,[dP/dx]$ from Equation 7.31, and therefore $0 = -D_ek\,[dP/dx]$. The term dP/dx can be obtained by differentiating the general expression given in Equation 7.26:

$$\frac{dP}{dx} = \left[\frac{Qx}{D_ek}\right] + B \qquad (7.43)$$

But the boundary condition for the tight oxygen-impermeable contact lens is that $0 = -D_ek\,[dP/dx]$ at $x = L$. Since D_ek cannot be zero, $dP/dx = 0$. Equation 7.43 becomes

$$0 = \left[\frac{Qx}{D_ek}\right] + B \qquad (7.44)$$

and at $x = L$, by rearrangement

$$B = -\left[\frac{QL}{D_ek}\right] \qquad (7.45)$$

Substituting this value for B (while $C = 55$ mmHg) into Equation 7.26 gives

$$P = \left[\frac{Qx^2}{2D_ek}\right] - \left[\frac{QLx}{D_ek}\right] + 55 \text{ mmHg} \qquad (7.46)$$

We will now examine Equations 7.42 and 7.46 together because they require a more detailed discussion of the physiological quantities that appear as constants, particularly the oxygen consumption rate Q.

It must be emphasized that mathematics does not always lead to a useful description of the real world. For example, Figures 7.10 and 7.11 show negative values of oxygen tension in profiles calculated for the boundary conditions of the nitrogen goggle experiments. Negative values arise in Figure 7.10 if the group $[Qx^2/2D_e k + 55 \text{ mmHg}]$ is less than $([QL/2D_e k] + [55 \text{ mmHg/L}]x)$, and the negative values seen in Figure 7.11 occur when $[Qx^2/2D_e k + 55 \text{ mmHg}]$ is less than $[QLx/2D_e k]$. Since negative oxygen tensions cannot exist in reality, we must find the source of these unreal tensions.

There are two methods for avoiding a mathematically derived oxygen tension profile with negative values. We can first maintain the argument that the oxygen consumption rate Q is independent of the oxygen tension in the tissue, and then accept a result that shows a completely anoxic zone in which the cells of the cornea have switched to anerobic metabolism or have died. No oxygen diffuses through this tissue beyond a point identified as x_c. Recall this is a model one-layer cornea that receives oxygen across its posterior surface but with no oxygen at $x = L$. This is shown graphically in Figure 7.12.

For the nitrogen goggle experiment we then have the following boundary conditions:

$$x = 0, P = 55 \text{ mmHg}$$
$$x = x_c, P = 0 \text{ mmHg} \qquad (7.47)$$
$$x = x_c, \frac{dP}{dx} = 0$$

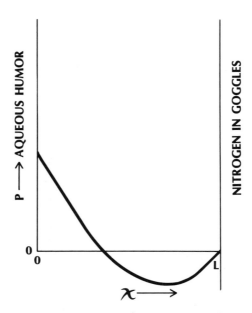

Figure 7.10 An unrealistic representation of oxygen tension in a cornea covered by goggles in which there is pure nitrogen. There is no physical meaning to the negative oxygen tension shown by the profile.

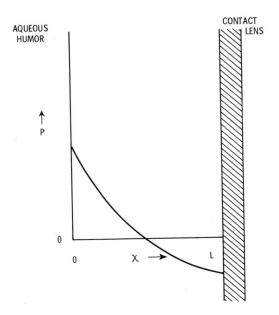

Figure 7.11 An unrealistic representation of oxygen tension in a cornea covered by a gas-impermeable contact lens. There is no physical meaning to negative oxygen tension.

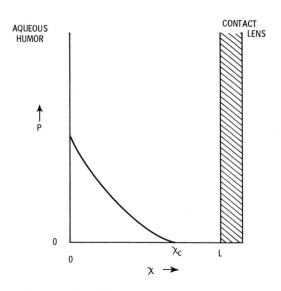

Figure 7.12 A true representation of oxygen tension in a cornea covered by a gas-impermeable contact lens. The oxygen tension becomes zero at X_c, and the slope of the profile is also zero at this point.

Note that we do not know x_c. But since we have an extra boundary condition we can proceed to evaluate B and C in Equation 7.26 even if the condition at x_c is not specified.

We again find that $C = 55$ mmHg as above. If we also substitute the second boundary condition from Equation 7.47 into Equation 7.26 we obtain

$$0 = \left[\frac{Qx_c^2}{2D_ek}\right] + Bx_c + 55 \text{ mmHg} \tag{7.48}$$

To use the third boundary condition from Equation 7.47 we first differentiate Equation 7.26:

$$\frac{dP}{dx} = \left[\frac{Qx}{D_ek}\right] + B \tag{7.49}$$

and then substitute the third boundary condition

$$0 = \left[\frac{Qx_c}{D_ek}\right] + B \tag{7.50}$$

Equations 7.48 and 7.50 are two simultaneous equations with the two unknowns: B and x_c. When solved, this set of equations gives

$$B = -\left[110 \text{ mmHg} \frac{Q}{D_ek}\right]^{1/2} \tag{7.51}$$

and

$$x_c = \left[110 \text{ mmHg} \frac{D_ek}{Q}\right]^{1/2} \tag{7.52}$$

which locates x_c in the model cornea. The equation for the oxygen tension profile can now be written for the case when oxygen enters the cornea only from the posterior surface:

$$P = \left[\frac{Qx^2}{2D_ek}\right] - x\left[110 \text{ mmHg} \frac{Q}{D_ek}\right]^{1/2} + 55 \text{ mmHg} \tag{7.53}$$

Equation 7.53 is also applicable for the case when the corneal anterior surface is covered by a tight oxygen-impermeable contact lens because it was derived without stating the condition at $x = L$. All that is required is that oxygen enters the cornea only at $x = 0$.

There is a second and perhaps physiologically more satisfactory method for eliminating unrealistic negative values for oxygen tensions in calculated profiles. In studies on single-cell organisms or suspensions of tissue cells, it is noted that oxygen consumption remains independent of oxygen tension until the tension is reduced to about 20 mmHg. There is then a sharp drop in the oxygen consumption rate. The differential equation for oxygen diffusion in the cornea when the cellular consumption rate is a function of oxygen tension becomes

$$\frac{d^2P}{dx^2} = \frac{Q(P)}{D_ek} \tag{7.54}$$

Equation 7.54 is applied only to those portions of the cornea where the oxygen tension has fallen below the value where oxygen consumption is independent of oxygen tension. The mathematical methods for deriving oxygen tension profiles under these conditions is beyond the scope of this text but is available in the literature (Fatt 1968b; Fatt et al. 1969).

The Case of the Tight Gas-Permeable Contact Lens

This situation applies primarily to the hydrogel contact lens, where tear exchange is minimal (Wagner et al. 1980). It might also apply to a tightly fitted rigid gas-permeable contact lens. Similarly, there is some evidence to suggest that tear exchange is depressed for all contact lenses worn under closed-eye (i.e., extended-wear) conditions.

Oxygen tension profiles can be calculated here by a simple extension of the methods explained earlier. The basic differential equation describing oxygen tension in our hypothetical one-layer cornea, Equation 7.26, is still applicable, as long as we assume that oxygen consumption is independent of oxygen tension. When another layer is placed on the cornea, a similar equation will apply to this new layer, but with different constants. Therefore, Equation 7.26 can be rewritten

$$P_{cl} = \left[\frac{Q}{2Dk'}\right]_{cl} x^2 + [B'x] + C' \tag{7.55}$$

where the primed quantities are specifically for the contact lens. P_{cl} is similarly the oxygen tension at any point along the x dimension in the contact lens. As the contact lens material is assumed to be inert, that is, free of oxygen-consuming or oxygen-producing cells (or microorganisms), Q is zero and Equation 7.55 becomes

$$P_{cl} = B'x + C' \tag{7.56}$$

We must now solve two equations with four undetermined constants, namely Equations 7.26 and 7.56 with constants B, C, B', and C'. This will require that we know the oxygen tension or oxygen tension gradient at four values of x.

At the interface between the cornea and the contact lens ($x = L$), there must be a continuity of oxygen flux. This boundary is a mathematically defined plane and has no volume itself. Therefore, whatever oxygen enters this boundary must also leave it. Stated mathematically, the condition at this boundary between cornea and lens is $j_c = j_{cl}$ at $x = L$. The subscripts c and cl indicate cornea and contact lens, respectively. From the definition of flux in Equation 7.9 and Henry's law we can rewrite this boundary condition as: $x = L$, $(-D_ek)_c (dP/dx)_c = (-Dk)_{cl} (dP/dx)_{cl}$ or

$$x = L, \left(\frac{dP}{dx}\right)_c = S \left(\frac{dP}{dx}\right)_{cl} \tag{7.57}$$

where $S = (-Dk)_{cl}/(-D_ek)_c$

Another condition at $x = L$ is that $P_c = P_{cl}$. This condition arises from our definition of P as oxygen tension. From the physical chemist's point of view, oxygen tension is the chemical activity of the oxygen dissolved in the cornea and contact lens. Chemical activity must be equal across a mathematical boundary of no thickness or there would be an infinite gradient; that is, as the thickness of the boundary Δx approaches zero, so must ΔP. If this were not true, there would be a jump in P at the boundary, and such a jump would have $dP/dx = $ infinity and lead to the prediction of an infinite flux, obviously an impossibility. Oxygen tension must therefore be equal on both sides of this boundary.

The oxygen tension at the anterior surface of the contact lens (at $x = L'$) is 155 mmHg if the eye is open (and at sea level). If the eye is closed, the oxygen tension at the anterior surface of the lens should be that of the palpebral conjunctiva, 55 mmHg as discussed above. To allow use of either situation in the final equation, we will say

$$x = L', P = P_L' \tag{7.58}$$

and insert the value of P_L, as indicated when we wish to apply the result to either the case of an open or closed eye.

We know that the oxygen tension of the aqueous humor boundary is 55 mmHg as discussed above, so that $P = 55$ mmHg at $x = 0$; therefore, as above, C is 55 mmHg. This leaves us only B, B', and C' to evaluate.

Equations 7.26 and 7.56 must give the same value for P at the boundary of the contact lens and cornea, $x = L$; therefore

$$\left[\frac{Q}{2D_e k}\right]_c L^2 + BL + 55 \text{ mmHg} = B'L + C' \tag{7.59}$$

When we evaluate and equate the fluxes at $x = L$ we get

$$QL + B(D_e k)_c = B'(Dk)_{cl} \tag{7.60}$$

At $x = L'$ we have

$$P_{L'} = B'L' + C' \tag{7.61}$$

Equations 7.59, 7.60, and 7.61 form a set of three simultaneous equations with three unknowns (B, B', and C') and are solved to give

$$B = \frac{Q(L - L')L - (Q(D_e k)_{cl} L^2 / 2(D_e k)_c) - 55(D_e k)_{cl} + P_{L'}(D_e k)_{cl}}{L(D_e k)_{cl} - (D_e k)_c (L - L')} \tag{7.62}$$

$$B' = \frac{QL}{(D_e k)_{cl}} \tag{7.63}$$

$$+\frac{(D_e k)_c}{(D_e k)_{cl}} \frac{Q(L - L')L - (Q(D_e k)_{cl} L^2 / 2(D_e k)_c) - 55(D_e k)_{cl} + P_{L'}(D_e k)_{cl}}{L(D_e k)_{cl} - (D_e k)_c (L - L')}$$

$$C' = P_{L'} - \frac{QLL'}{(D_e k)_{cl}} \tag{7.64}$$

$$+ \frac{(D_e k)_c L'}{(D_e k)_{cl}} \frac{Q(L - L')L - (Q(D_e k)_{cl} L^2 / 2(D_e k)_c) - 55(D_e k)_{cl} + P_{L'} (D_e k)_{cl}}{L(D_e k)_{cl} - (D_e k)_c (L - L')}$$

If numerical values are available for all the terms on the right-hand sides of Equations 7.62, 7.63, and 7.64, the constants B, B', and C' can be evaluated and oxygen tension profiles then drawn as shown in Figure 7.13.

The procedure described above (for obtaining oxygen tension profiles in the hypothetical one-layer cornea) is exact but cumbersome. Also, it has the weakness of assuming that the cornea, which is really multilayered, can be approximated by a homogenous single-tissue layer with properties that are an average of the individual layer properties, and that the oxygen consumption rate is independent of oxygen tension. Furthermore, because of the discussion of the COT above, an oxygen tension value of specific interest is that of the tear–cornea boundary just under a contact lens.

Oxygen Tension at the Corneal Surface

Fatt and St Helen (1971) suggested a simplified approach to estimate the oxygen tension at the anterior corneal surface using the results of Fatt, Bieber, and Pye (1969), who showed that the oxygen flux into the anterior surface of the (multilayered) cornea could be expressed as

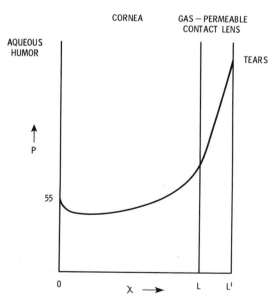

Figure 7.13 Oxygen tension in a cornea covered by a gas-permeable contact lens.

$$j_c = \alpha \, P_L{}^{\beta} \tag{7.65}$$

Values for the constants α and β in Equation 7.65 have been developed from Figure 9 of Fatt, Bieber, and Pye (1969) and the data of Haberich (1966) (Fatt 1969b). α is taken as 0.24×10^{-6} ml O_2/cm^2 sec (mmHg)$^{1/2}$ (or 0.864 μl O_2/cm^2 hour mmHg) and β as 1/2. This oxygen flux relationship is shown by the dashed curve in Figure 7.14.

As the contact lens and cornea are joined at a mathematical plane, oxygen that enters the cornea at the anterior surface must have come through the gas-permeable contact lens on the eye, or mathematically $j_c = j_{cl}$. The equation for oxygen flux through the contact lens is

$$j_{cl} = \left(\frac{Dk}{L'}\right) \, cl \, (P_{L'} - P_L) \tag{7.66}$$

where Dk/L is the oxygen transmissibility of the contact lens at ocular temperature. Equations 7.65 and 7.66 may therefore be equated, giving

$$\alpha \, P_L{}^{\beta} = \left(\frac{Dk}{L'}\right) \, _{cl} (P_{L'} - P_L) \tag{7.67}$$

To test the continued applicability of Equation 7.65 with recent data, we can examine the data of Weissman and co-workers (1988) who found that 8 hours' wear of hydrogel contact lenses of known Dk/L values under open-eye conditions

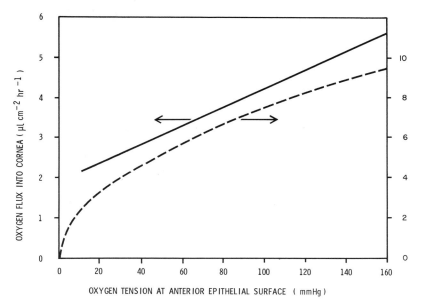

Figure 7.14 Oxygen flux into a cornea as a function of oxygen tension at the anterior epithelial surface. ----, from the earlier calculations of Fatt and St. Helen (1971); —, from the more recent data of Fatt, Freeman, and Lin (1974).

induced average corneal swelling as shown in Table 7.3. The oxygen tension expected under the contact lenses was estimated from Figure 7.8. Equation 7.66 can then be used to give the j_{cl}, which must equal j_c. Now we have several paired j_{cl} and P_L values. We can produce similar data for j_c from the same P_L values by Equation 7.65. By inspection, the pairs of j values produced are very similar and also consistent with the results of both Hill and Fatt (1963b) and Larke and associates (1981).

Equation 7.67 may be solved for P_L, the oxygen tension in the tear layer between the contact lens and the cornea, by the quadratic formula after squaring both sides. Given the properties of the covering contact lens (its Dk/L value), the oxygen tension at the anterior surface of the lens (P_L equals 155 mmHg if the eye is open or 55 mmHg if the eye is closed), and assuming that the flux into the cornea is predicted by $j_c = \alpha P^\beta$, the oxygen tension under the lens may be calculated. The dashed line in Figure 7.15 was produced from Equation 7.67 assuming α and β are constants as described above. It is assumed also that blinking does not affect these results for the open eye because (1) this lens is fitted to disallow any tear exchange, and (2) the time that the eye is covered by the lid is too small to perturb the steady-state condition. Likewise, the closed-eye solution is for an eye that has been closed long enough to reach steady state. This would be on the order of 5 minutes.

Alternatively, Fatt, Freeman, and Lin (1974) have used the oxygen consumption data of Freeman (1972) and the corneal $D_e k$ values of Freeman and Fatt (1972) to calculate oxygen flux at the anterior surface of a multilayered cornea. Their results are shown by the solid line in Figure 7.14. This differs from the earlier result of Fatt, Bieber, and Pye (1969) in several aspects. First, the Fatt, Freeman, and Lin (1974) relationship is linear with respect to P_L, and the equation for flux is therefore written

$$j_c = aP_L + b \qquad (7.68)$$

where a and b are new constants. Second, the Fatt, Freeman, and Lin (1974) relationship does not yield zero flux for zero oxygen tension as does the Fatt, Bieber, and Pye (1969) line. Note that the solid line in Figure 7.14 is *not* drawn below 10 mmHg. Fatt, Freeman, and Lin (1974) used oxygen consumption rates

Table 7.3 Anterior Surface Corneal Oxygen Flux (j) Predicted from Corneal Swelling Associated with 8 Hours of Open-Eye Hydrogel Contact Lens Wear* Compared to that Predicted by $j_c = \alpha P^{1/2}$

Dk/L (cm ml O_2 sec ml mmHg)	% Cornea Swelling (Mean; N = 5)	%O_2	P_L (mmHg) (from Figure 7.8)	j_{cl}	j_c (μl O_2/cm_2 hour)
20×10^{-9}	1.2	6.0	44	8.0	5.7
12×10^{-9}	1.8	4.0	30	5.4	4.7
6.8×10^{-9}	2.2	2.5	19	3.3	3.8

*Lenses of measured Dk/L values as shown from Weissman et al. 1988.

for the epithelium and endothelium that were independent of oxygen tension; as this is not believed to be true for most living cells and is unlikely in these cellular layers, the line is not extended into this doubtful region. Third, the flux values from the Fatt, Freeman, and Lin (1974) relationship are quantitatively less than those of Fatt, Bieber, and Pye (1969) at all oxygen tensions.

When Equations 7.66 and 7.68 are equated and a consistent set of units are used, the result is

$$\left(\frac{Dk}{L}\right)_{cl} = \frac{[(0.5 \times 10^{-6}) + (0.66 \times 10^{-6})P_L]}{(P_{L'} - P_L)} \qquad (7.69)$$

where Dk/L will be in cm ml O_2/sec ml mmHg, when P_L' and P_L are in mmHg. The solid lines in Figure 7.15 show the oxygen tension under an oxygen-permeable contact lens, with no tear exchange, predicted by use of Equation 7.69 to compare with the dashed lines calculated from Equation 7.67; note that the two methods do not predict vastly different results.

We can now use Figure 7.15 to examine the effect of an oxygen-permeable contact lens, rigid or hydrogel, with no tear exchange, on anterior corneal surface oxygen tension. Let us assume that the eye is covered by a hydrogel contact lens

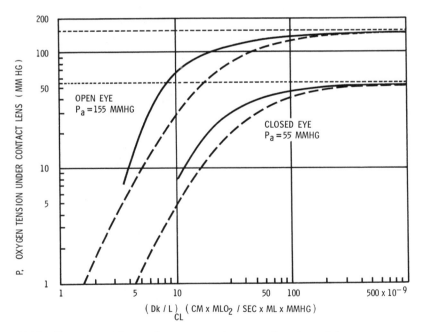

Figure 7.15 Oxygen tension under a contact lens as a function of the oxygen transmissibility of the lens. ----, from the earlier calculations of Fatt and St. Helen (1971); —, from the more recent data of Fatt, Freeman, and Lin (1974). (From Fatt I [1977]: A rational method for the design of gas-permeable soft contact lenses. The Optician [London] 173 [4470]:10–15.)

with $Dk = 9 \times 10^{-11}$ cm^2 ml O$_2$/sec ml mmHg and thickness 0.2 mm. This is similar to the early first-generation lenses made from hydroxyethylmethacrylate (HEMA) with a 38% water content. The value of Dk/L is then 4.5×10^{-9} cm ml O$_2$/sec ml mmHg. For the open eye, Figure 7.15 indicates P_L will be about 10 mmHg by either the solid or dashed line. We remember that this meets the original COT proposed by Polse and Mandell (1970), but as we now believe that the COT may be greater we would predict some corneal swelling would be caused by such a lens. Sleeping with this lens on the eye will produce an oxygen tension at the corneal surface of about 1 mmHg, which is quite unacceptable.

Assume that the lens is now made thinner: 0.09 mm. The Dk/L value increases to 10×10^{-9} cm ml O$_2$/sec ml mmHg. Open-eye conditions suggest that P_L will increase to 30 to 70 mmHg, which is much more acceptable. This was the basis for the development of the "ultrathin" soft lens in the early 1980s. P_L for the closed eye, however, is still below 10 mmHg.

The highest Dk currently available for a hydrogel material is about 35×10^{-11} cm^2 ml O$_2$/sec ml mmHg (80% water); making a lens from this material 0.14 mm thick would result in a Dk/L of 25×10^{-9}, leading to a predicted P_L of 80 to 120 mmHg under open-eye conditions, and 20 to 35 mmHg under closed-eye conditions. This is undoubtedly adequate for the open eye but may not be adequate for all eyes under closed-eye conditions; recall the variability of corneal responses to hypoxia indicated in Figure 7.8 and in the data of Larke and co-workers (1981).

By monitoring human subjects wearing contact lenses, Holden and Mertz (1984) determined that a Dk/L value of 24×10^{-9} precluded corneal swelling under open-eye conditions; this figure is consistent with the results of a similar study by Weissman and associates (1988). For closed-eye conditions, Holden and Mertz (1984) found a Dk/L value of 87×10^{-9} was needed, and O'Neal and colleagues (1984) found a value of 75×10^{-9}.

The Case of the Gas-Impermeable Contact Lenses with Tear Pumping

The original "hard" contact lenses were made from Plexiglass, or Lucite (polymethylmethacrylate, or PMMA). This plastic allows good optics and machines well, but it is essentially impermeable to oxygen. Largely because of the work described above concerning the oxygen requirements of the cornea, this plastic has fallen out of clinical favor. Yet we shall consider it here (1) for historical reasons and (2) because it allows us to explore the mathematics describing tear exchange under contact lenses.

Lenses made from PMMA can be tolerated on the cornea only because they move with each blink, thereby bringing fresh, oxygenated tears to the cornea every few seconds. Each contact lens–cornea relationship captures a certain volume of tears between the adjacent surfaces, but it is unlikely that the total volume will be exchanged with each blink (this would be an efficiency of 100%). Cuklanz and Hill (1969) calculated that a well-fitted rigid lens will exchange about 20% of the tear volume per blink (for comparison, Wagner and co-workers [1980] found that hydrogel lenses only exchange about 1% to 2% of their tear layers per blink, regardless of fitting relationship). Oxygen used by the cornea from the tears under the contact lens is not replaced between blinks when gas-impermeable lenses are worn. As we noted above, we would predict that a cornea will swell if these blinks did not bring enough air-saturated tears underneath the covering lens to keep the oxygen tension in the trapped tear layer above 40 to 70 mmHg.

Fatt (1969b) and Cuklanz and Hill (1969) developed a quantitative description of oxygen movement through the tear film under an oxygen-*impermeable* contact lens with blinking. This work was later expanded to oxygen-*permeable* lenses (Fatt and Lin 1976; Fatt and Liu 1984). The movement of oxygen into the cornea is given by Equation 7.9, but assuming that the oxygen tension in the tears under the lens falls slowly or through only a small range so that the oxygen tension profile across the cornea is never very far from the steady state allows use of either Equation 7.65 or 7.68 to describe the movement of oxygen into the cornea. Fatt (1969b) chose to use Equation 7.65 because it was all that was available at the time, but it is also easier to manipulate mathematically, extends to lower oxygen tensions, and gives a more conservative estimate of oxygen tension. We have shown above that this relationship still appears consistent with modern data. Between blinks, the consumed oxygen comes only from the tear layer trapped under the contact lens. Depletion of oxygen from this space (between the lens back surface and the anterior cornea) must also equal $-(Vk/a)\,(dP/dt)$, where V is the volume of tears beneath the contact lens, k the oxygen solubility of the tear film, and a the area of corneal surface covered; dP/dt is the change in oxygen pressure P over time t, as discussed above. The negative sign denotes the depletion process. Therefore

$$\alpha P^{1/2} = -\frac{Vk}{a}\frac{dP}{dt} \tag{7.70}$$

Equation 7.70 states that the oxygen flux into the cornea is a power function of the oxygen tension under the lens. The assumption that the oxygen tension profile across the cornea is always at or near the steady state will exaggerate the effect of blinking, and the resulting analysis to follow will therefore present the most pessimistic case for oxygen supply by tear exchange.

Equation 7.70 can be written in integral form as

$$\int_0^{\Delta t} dt = -\frac{Vk}{a\alpha}\int_{P_a}^{P_1}\frac{dP}{P^{1/2}} \tag{7.71}$$

Here Δt is the time between insertion of the contact lens onto the cornea and the first blink. Later blinks will be at $2 \times \Delta t$, $3 \times \Delta t$, $4 \times \Delta t \dots n \times \Delta t$, where Δt is the time interval between blinks. P_a is the oxygen tension in the incoming tear fluid, assumed to be saturated with air under open-eye conditions. P_1 is the oxygen tension in the trapped tears just before the first blink. Integration of Equation 7.71 gives

$$\Delta t = -\frac{2Vk}{a\alpha}(P_1^{1/2} - P_a^{1/2}) \tag{7.72}$$

All terms in Equation 7.72 are known or can be set except P_1, so we can evaluate this relationship for P_1.

At Δt, a blink takes place that will cause an exchange of tears. We set the fraction of tear volume exchanged as $1 - f$, where f is the fraction that remains behind. The volume of dissolved oxygen in the reservoir just before the blink is given by

$$V_1 = kVP_1 \tag{7.73}$$

After the blink, the dissolved oxygen remaining in the *unexchanged* tears is

$$V_{1-} = fkVP_1 \tag{7.74}$$

and the amount of oxygen *brought in* by the fresh tears is

$$V_{1+} = (1 - f)kVP_a \tag{7.75}$$

The new total oxygen volume is therefore

$$V_{1-} + V_{1+} = fkVP_1 + (1 - f)kVP_a \tag{7.76}$$

The oxygen tension under the lens now rises to P_2, given by

$$P_2 = \left(\frac{V_{1-} + V_{1+}}{Vk}\right) \tag{7.77}$$

Combining Equations 7.76 and 7.77 gives

$$P_2 = fP_1 + (1 - f)P_a \tag{7.78}$$

If f is known, P_2 may now be calculated from Equation 7.78. Equation 7.72 is now used to determine the drop in P to P_3 over the second interblink period:

$$\Delta t = -\left(\frac{2Vk}{a\alpha}\right)(P_3^{1/2} - P_2^{1/2}) \tag{7.79}$$

Again, all terms in Equation 7.79 are known except P_3, so P_3 may be calculated.

After the next blink, the oxygen tension under the lens will jump to P_4 and then slowly decline to P_5 in a similar manner, and it will reach P_5 at $3\Delta t$. To calculate P_4, P_5, and subsequent values of P we proceed as above.

Figure 7.16 was constructed by this process to show the periodically changing oxygen tension under a lens of known parameters. The average oxygen tension under the lens will continue to fall until the replenishment of oxygen by a blink is just equal to the amount consumed by the cornea during the same time period. All further blinks will then give oxygen tensions oscillating about a fixed average. It is this condition that is of most interest because a calculation based on the procedure given above, and using the parameters to be given next, shows that this steady oscillation is reached after about five blinks. Therefore, for all periods of contact lens wear of greater than about one-half minute, the steady oscillating condition will be reached.

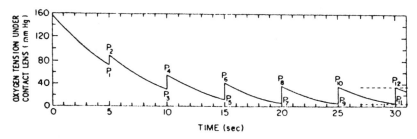

Figure 7.16 Oxygen tension under a contact lens as a function of time. Lens was inserted at $t = 0$; blink period is 5 seconds. The fractional tear volume replaced by a blink is 0.2, and the equivalent reservoir thickness is $0.35 \times 10^-$ cm. (From Fatt I [1969]: Oxygen tension under a contact lens during blinking. Am. J. Optom. 46:654–661.)

At the nth blink, integration of Equation 7.71 leads to

$$\Delta t = - \left(\frac{2Vk}{a\alpha}\right) (P_{n+1}^{1/2} - P_n^{1/2}) \tag{7.80}$$

The method above to calculate P_2 applies here and yields

$$P_{n+1} = fP_n + (1 - f)P_a \tag{7.81}$$

At steady state, the oscillation of oxygen tension under the lens will give an average that is constant with time. This means that the increases and decreases in oxygen tension will be the same with all subsequent blinks. Under this condition

$$P_n = P_{n+2} \tag{7.82}$$

Grouping Equations 7.80, 7.81, and 7.82 yields

$$P_{n+1}^{1/2} = \left(\frac{\Delta ta\alpha}{2Vk}\right) \left[fP_{n+1} + (1-f)P_a\right]^{1/2} \tag{7.83}$$

Solving Equation 7.83 for P_{n+1} gives the *minimum* oxygen tension under the lens at steady state. Equation 7.81 may also be solved for P_n to give the *maximum* oxygen tension for the steady-state situation.

The normal human blinking rate of 12/minute gives a Δt of 5 seconds to be used in Equation 7.72. Cuklanz and Hill (1968) give a value of 12×10^{-3} µl O_2 for VkP_a. Since P_a and k are known (155 mmHg and 4.4×10^{-5} ml O_2/ml tears mmHg, respectively), V can be calculated and is found to be 1.76×10^{-3} ml. Cuklanz and Hill (1968) also give a as 0.5 cm^2 for a normal rigid contact lens. V/a is then an equivalent thickness of the reservoir under the lens and is found to be 0.35×10^{-2} cm (35 µm). The values for the terms α and β have been discussed above. Equation 7.83 becomes

$$\Delta t = 5 \text{ sec} = -1.28 (P_1^{1/2} - 12.4) \tag{7.84}$$

Solving Equation 7.83 results in $P_1 = 72$ mmHg; this is the oxygen tension left under the contact lens after the first 5 seconds of wear and just prior to the first blink. The drop in P from $\Delta t = 0$ to $\Delta t = 5$ can be calculated from Equation 7.84 by using a series of values for Δt in this range. This curve is shown by the drop in oxygen tension from 160 to 72 mmHg in Figure 7.16.

Cuklanz and Hill (1968) found that the fraction of tear reservoir exchanged per blink was 0.2, and this was later confirmed by Hayashi (1977). The term f is therefore 0.8 and $1 - f$ is 0.2. P_2 can therefore be calculated from Equation 7.81 and is found to be 88.5 mmHg. This process was carried out for six blinks, and the results are shown in Figure 7.16. The final maximum and minimum oscillation values are shown by the short dashed lines to the right of this figure, ranging from 5 to 35 mmHg, with a mean of about 17 mmHg. It is clear that the system is operating in a steady oscillating state after the first four or five blinks.

Crossplotting these final maximum and minimum values while allowing the fractional tear volume replaced to vary between zero (the "tight" fit) and 0.5 (50% of the tears exchanged per blink) gives the graph shown in Figure 7.17. The dashed line here is the average oxygen tension predicted to be under the lens when the "steady-state" oscillation has been reached after about five blinks. Note that the mean oxygen tension value is less than 20 mmHg for a fractional exchange of 0.2. The current literature suggests this value is insufficient to maintain normal corneal physiology and will result in swelling and other disturbances. Increasing the fraction exchanged to 0.4 will increase the average oxygen tension under the lens to more than 40 mmHg, however, which might be adequate.

Figure 7.18 shows these results for a lens reservoir with an equivalent thickness that has been doubled to 0.70×10^{-2} cm (70 μm); note that here a fractional

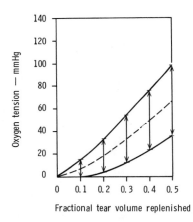

Fractional tear volume replenished

Figure 7.17 Steady-state oscillation of oxygen tension under a contact lens as a function of fractional tear volume replaced by a blink. The ratio, blink period to equivalent reservoir thickness, is 1430 sec/cm. →, the range of oxygen tension oscillation; ----, the time–average oxygen tension under the lens. (From Fatt I [1969]: Oxygen tension under a contact lens during blinking. Am. J. Optom. 46:654–661.)

replenishment rate of 0.2 will result in an average oxygen tension of about 40 mmHg under the lens. Figure 7.19 shows the results of the same calculations for a reservoir halved to 0.175×10^{-2} cm (17.5 μm). No oxygen is maintained under the lens under the latter conditions at the end of the interblink period unless the fractional replenishment rate is greater than 0.3. To obtain an average oxygen tension under the lens greater than 40 mmHg it is necessary to raise $1 - f$ to 0.5.

It is of interest to note that the time between blinks (Δt) is divided by V/a in Equation 7.83. This means that Figures 7.17, 7.18, and 7.19 are really for a combination of blink times and equivalent reservoir thicknesses. For example, in Figure 7.17, Δt/thickness is 1430 sec/cm; in Figure 7.18 this ratio is 715 sec/cm; and in Figure 7.19 it is 2145 sec/cm. Any blink time divided by equivalent reservoir thickness that will equal 1430 sec/cm will give the curves shown in Figure 7.17. Figures 7.17, 7.18, and 7.19 also show that, for a given $\Delta t\, a/V$, the average oxygen tension under the lens and the range of oscillation during blinking both increase as the fractional tear volume replenished increases. It appears that doubling the reservoir thickness doubles the average oxygen tension under the lens for a fixed blinking rate.

Figure 7.20 shows the time–average oxygen tension under a lens during blinking as a function of the ratio $\Delta t\, a/V$ for various values of f. The dashed portions of the curves (at high values of $\Delta t\, a/V$) show where the calculated minimum oxygen tension drops to zero between blinks. Figure 7.20 shows that the effects of changes in blinking rate and reservoir volume are important only for $\Delta t\, a/V$ less than 1500 sec/cm; above this value the curves are almost flat. A patient who is trained to improve his blinking and changes his $\Delta t\, a/V$ from 2500 to 1500

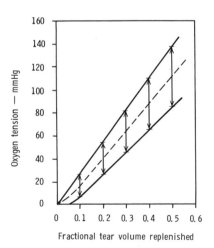

Figure 7.18 Steady-state oscillation of oxygen tension under a contact lens is a function of fractional tear volume replaced by a blink. Ratio, blink period to equivalent reservoir thickness, is 715 sec/cm. →, the range of oxygen tension oscillation; ----, the time–average oxygen tension under the lens. (From Fatt I [1969]: Oxygen tension under a contact lens during blinking. *Am. J. Optom.* 46:654–661.)

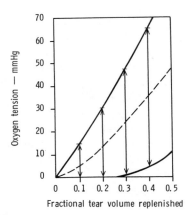

Figure 7.19 Steady-state oscillation of oxygen tension under a contact lens as a function of fractional tear volume replaced by a blink. The ratio, blink period to equivalent reservoir thickness, is 2145 sec/cm. →, the range of oxygen tension oscillation; ----, the time–average oxygen tension under the lens. (From Fatt I [1969]: Oxygen tension under a contact lens during blinking. Am. J. Optom. 46:654−661.)

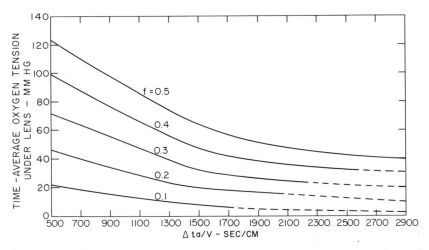

Figure 7.20 Time–average oxygen tension under a contact lens as a function of the ratio $\Delta t\, a/V$ for various values of the fractional volume of tear fluid replenished at a blink. ----, for values of the parameters where oxygen tension under the lens falls to zero between blinks. Numbers on curves are fractional volume of tear fluid under lens replenished at a blink. (From Fatt I [1969]: Oxygen tension under a contact lens during blinking. Am. J. Optom. 46:654−661.)

sec/cm will achieve almost no improvement in oxygen resupply. On the other hand, increasing the fractional replacement volume from 0.1 to 0.3, especially if $\Delta t\ a/V$ is below 1500 sec/cm, may have a substantial effect.

The mathematical procedure described above is based on too many poorly known properties of the cornea–contact lens system to be accepted without verification. An experiment was therefore made to obtain such verification.

Direct measurement of oxygen tension under a contact lens is possible by attaching a polarographic oxygen electrode to the center of the lens. The arrangement used by Fatt and Hill (1970) is shown in Figure 7.21. The data for two experimental lenses and test cornea systems are given in Table 7.4; reservoir

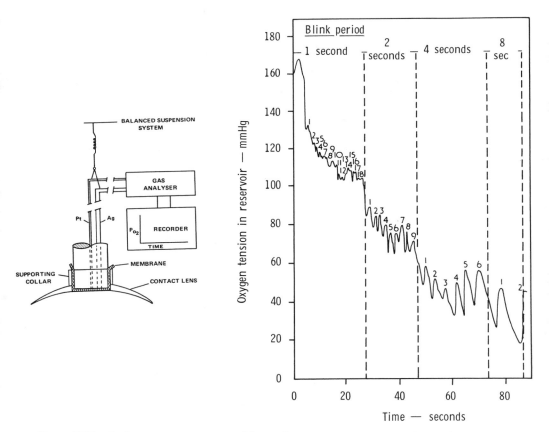

Figure 7.21 *Left,* oxygen sensor assembly used to measure oxygen tension under a contact lens during blinking. The platinum (Pt) and silver (Ag) wires form the sensor electrodes. The *Gas Analyzer* is an electronic device to convert sensor current to a signal that will operate the recorder. *Right,* oxygen tension recorded from the tear reservoir between a human cornea and a contact lens of System 1 (Table 7.4). (From Fatt I, Hill RM [1970]: Oxygen tension under a contact lens during blinking—a comparison of theory and experimental observation. Am. J. Optom. 47:50–55.)

volumes were obtained by direct measurement, as described by Cuklanz and Hill (1968). These volumes are considerably larger than would be predicted (by the method of Cuklanz and Hill [1968] from the lens and corneal curvatures) because the lens vault fitted with the flat-ended oxygen sensor deviates from the spherical geometry used in their model. The addition of the oxygen sensor increases the tear volume under the lens.

Each lens–electrode system, shown in Figure 7.21, was suspended so that it was as near weightless as possible on the human eye (i.e., approaching the weight of the unaltered lens at 20 mg). Since this suspension arrangement could only be operated with the subject in the supine position, the results must be restricted to this condition.

Figure 7.21 also shows the time course of oxygen tension in the tear reservoir of System 1 when operated at selected blink frequencies as shown. Figure 7.22 shows similar data for System 2.

Fatt's (1969b) theoretical model, described above, predicts that the decline in oxygen tension under a lens will be a function of the blink frequency, tear reservoir volume, and fractional replacement of tears under the lens at each blink. Figure 7.23 presents these predictions, redrawn from Figure 7.20, for the range of experimental data generated by Systems 1 and 2. The open circles in this figure represent the actual data found for System 1, and the crosses are for System 2; over most of the experimental range these data suggest that the replenishment factor is slightly below 0.2 (0.18 will be used below). Interpolation of these results by use of Figures 7.17, 7.18, and 7.19 gives oxygen tension values for comparison with those actually found in Systems 1 and 2, and these data are shown in Table 7.5.

The comparison of observed data with theoretical prediction presented in Figure 7.23 and Table 7.5 shows that the experimental average oxygen tension data found by Systems 1 and 2 follow very closely the theoretical predictions for the average and range of oxygen tension under a contact lens with a stable blinking rate.

Unfortunately, Figure 7.23 is not of great clinical value because the maximum of the group $\Delta t\, a/V$ is not realistic for well-fitted contact lenses. An 8.0-mm

Table 7.4 Physical Properties of Lens-Electrode Systems*

Lens Total Diameter (mm)	Base Curve Radius (mm)	Corneal Radii (mm)	Reservoir Volume (μl)	a/V_1 (cm^{-1})
System 1				
10.0	7.94	7.95 (180°) 7.76 (90°)	5.8	135.5
System 2				
8.0	7.94	7.95 (180°) 7.76 (90°)	7.5	67.0

*From Fatt I, Hill RM (1970): Oxygen tension under a contact lens during blinking—a comparison of theory and experimental observation. Am. J. Optom. 47:50–55.

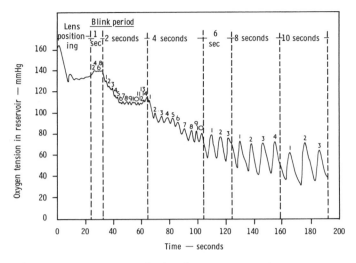

Figure 7.22 Same as Figure 7.21, *right,* but for System 2 (Table 7.4). (From Fatt I, Hill RM [1970]: Oxygen tension under a contact lens during blinking—a comparison of theory and experimental observation. Am. J. Optom. 47:50–55.)

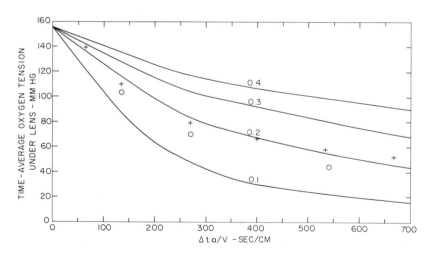

Figure 7.23 The time–average oxygen tension under a contact lens as a function of $\Delta t \ a/V$ and the fractional tear volume replenishment (marked on the curves). ○, experimental data points for System 1 (Table 7.4); ×, for System 2 (Table 7.4). (From Fatt I, Hill RM [1970]: Oxygen tension under a contact lens during blinking—a comparison of theory and experimental observation. J. Am. Optom. 47:50–55.)

Table 7.5 Experimental and Theoretical Oxygen Tensions for Lens–Electrode Systems on Human Eye*

Blink Period (seconds)	Δt Q/V (sec/cm)	Observed Stable Average Oxygen Tension (mmHg)	Observed Range of Oxygen Tension at Stability (mmHg)	Theoretical Oxygen Tensions for System with Fractional Tear Replenishment of 0.18 at Stability	
				Average (mmHg)	Range (mmHg)
System 1					
1	135	104	2	115	8
2	270	71	12	79	20
4	540	46	18	50	22
8	1080	31	30	25	30
System 2					
1	66.7	138	2	132	6
2	133	108	4	115	8
4	267	74	12	79	20
6	400	67	23	61	20
8	534	56	32	50	22
10	667	51	42	39	28

*From Fatt I, Hill RM (1970): Oxygen tension under a contact lens during blinking—a comparison of theory and experimental observation. Am. J. Optom. 47:50–55.

diameter rigid lens may have a tear reservoir as low as 0.2 μl; at a normal blink rate of 12 blinks/minute ($\Delta t = 5$ sec), $\Delta t\, a/V$ becomes 12,500 sec/cm. Figures 7.20 and 7.23 indicate that increasing the fractional tear replenishment rate is much more effective at increasing oxygen tension under an oxygen-impermeable lens than is either increasing blink rate or decreasing reservoir volume. However, oxygen-*permeable* rigid contact lenses have been available since about 1980, and this changes the clinical utilization of this information, as we will see below.

Before we move on to the case of oxygen-permeable contact lens with tear pumping, we should note another way to improve the oxygen tension under a contact lens. Polse and Mandell (1971) studied corneal swelling during wear of an impermeable contact lens when environmental oxygen tension was raised from normal room air (155 mmHg, or 21% O_2) to 600 mmHg (80%). Fatt (1971b) used the parameters of their test lens, assuming a fractional exchange rate of 0.1, to produce Figure 7.24. It shows the environmental oxygen tensions required to predict average oxygen tensions under such a lens of 5, 10, or 20 mmHg. We now know these values are all probably insufficient to preclude corneal swelling, but the data of Polse and Mandell (1971) are still of interest. Figure 7.25 is a crossplot of these data.

Polse and Mandell (1971) found that use of their contact lens caused 6.5% swelling when the oxygen tension of the external environment was 155 mmHg,

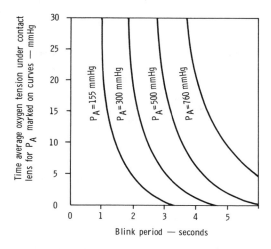

Figure 7.24 Time–average oxygen tension under a contact lens for various blink periods and oxygen tension (P_A) in the environment. (From Fatt I [1971]: Influence of hyperbaric environment on oxygen tension under a contact lens. Am. J. Optom. 48:109–112.)

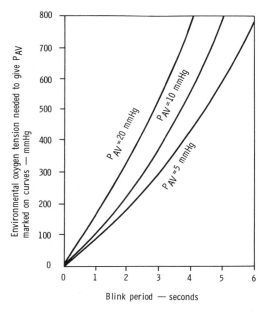

Figure 7.25 Environmental oxygen tension required to maintain a time–average oxygen tension (P_{AV}) of 5, 10, or 20 mmHg under a contact lens as a function of blink period. (From Fatt I [1971]: Influence of hyperbaric environment on oxygen tension under a contact lens. Am. J. Optom. 48:109–112.)

and decreasing levels of swelling were associated with increasing oxygen tensions (almost 6% at 300 mmHg, 2.5% at 450 mmHg, and 1.5% at 600 mmHg). Figure 7.8 allows conversion of these swelling data into expected oxygen tension values in the tear reservoir of about 0 mmHg, 8 mmHg, 20 mmHg, and 40 mmHg, respectively. Use of a time–average oxygen tension under the lens of 20 mmHg at an environmental oxygen tension of 450 mmHg (60% O_2) and Figures 7.24 and 7.25 suggests that this subject had a blink period of about 3 seconds if the tear replenishment rate was 0.1 as assumed in the calculations. Cuklanz and Hill (1969) observed mixing efficiencies of 0.09 to 0.13 for several different contact lenses.

The Case of the Oxygen-Permeable Contact Lens with Tear Pumping

It appears that the tear exchange under a hydrogel lens is insufficient to supply the cornea with much oxygen, even across a range of fitting relationships. Rigid gas-permeable contact lenses combine both the tear-pumping mechanism and diffusion to provide an oxygen supply to the cornea. The original rigid gas-permeable materials like cellulose acetate butyrate (CAB) and Polycon had low oxygen permeabilities (about 5 to 10×10^{-11} cm^2 ml O_2/sec ml mmHg, or about the same as 38% water content hydrogels), but more modern materials have Dk values of 40 to 100×10^{-11} cm^2 ml O_2/sec ml mmHg. Table 7.6 gives values for a large variety of materials. When diffusion of oxygen through the contact lens is combined with oxygen brought under the lens by tear exchange, a substantial improvement in oxygen supply may be achieved.

Fatt and Lin (1976) presented a mathematical analysis of the movement of oxygen to the cornea under a gas-permeable contact lens in the presence of tear pumping. The analysis uses a simple combination of Equations 7.67 and 7.70:

$$\left(\frac{Dk}{L}\right)_{cl} (P_a - P_L) - \alpha P_L^{1/2} = \left(\frac{Vk}{a}\right) \left(\frac{dP_L}{dt}\right) \tag{7.85}$$

Equation 7.85 says that the rate of oxygen supply to the tear film under the lens by diffusion ($Dk/L \times \Delta P$) less the rate of corneal oxygen consumption ($\alpha P_L^{1/2}$) must equal the rate of change in oxygen in the tear film under the lens. This equation clearly applies to the period of time between blinks. The oxygen tension increase in the tear film under the lens when a blink occurs is still given by Equation 7.78, and it is now a matter of making the same analysis as above from Equations 7.70 to 7.84, but in this instance Equation 7.85 is used in place of 7.70 as the starting point.

Figure 7.26 shows the results of these calculations for a contact lens with a Dk/L value of 18.8×10^{-9} cm ml O_2/sec ml mmHg, a blink period of 5 seconds, with tear film thickness set at 32 μm and a tear exchange fraction of 0.2. Note that this results in an average oxygen tension under the lens of about 70 mmHg. Reducing the fractional tear exchange to 0 reduces this to 60 mmHg, but making the lens impermeable while keeping the fractional tear exchange rate at 0.2 reduces the average oxygen tension under the lens to about 20 mmHg. It is clear

Table 7.6 List of Dk Values for Series of Modern Rigid Gas-Permeable Materials*

	Permeability and Relative Permeability at 35° C of Gas-Permeable Hard Materials			
(1) Material	(2) *Permeability*† @ 35° C *Without Edge Effect Correction*	(3) *Permeability* @ 35° C *with Edge Effect Correction*	(4) *Relative Permeability Without Edge Effect Correction*	(5) *Relative Permeability with Edge Effect Correction*
3M	95×10^{-11}	78×10^{-11}	100	100
Paraperm EW II	92	75	97	96
Optacryl Z	67	54	71	69
Alberta Supra B	66	53	69	68
Equalens	55	44	58	56
Optacryl EXT	54	43	57	55
Paraperm EW	49	39	52	50
Alberta N	40	31	42	40
Paraperm O₂ Plus	39	31	41	40
Alberta 3	36	28	38	36
Boston IV	24	18	25	23
Alberta 2	22	17	23	22
Paraperm O₂	18	14	19	18
Boston II	14	11	15	14

*From Fatt I, Rasson JE, Melpolder JB (1987): Measuring oxygen permeability of gas-permeable hard and hydrogel lenses and flat samples in air. Int. Contact Lens Clin. 14:389–401, 1987.
†Units of Permeability are (cm²/sec) (ml O_2/ml × mmHg).

that even modest amounts of oxygen permeability in a contact lens material will go a long way toward reducing corneal hypoxia regardless of tear exchange. Some comment is necessary concerning the choice of 32 μm as a tear layer thickness; this is clinically somewhat excessive, but it was chosen so that there would be an easily seen difference between situations where there is or is not tear pumping.

Figure 7.27 is a crossplot of similar calculations (from Fatt and Liu 1984) and shows how the average oxygen under a contact lens increases for increasing oxygen transmissibility with four fractional exchange rates between 0 and 0.20, with blink period held constant at 5 seconds and tear film thickness held constant at 20 μm. It is clear that increasing Dk/L from 10 to 15×10^{-9} is more effective at increasing oxygen tension in the tears than increasing the fractional replenishment rate from 0 to 0.15 for the same original Dk/L of 10×10^{-9}.

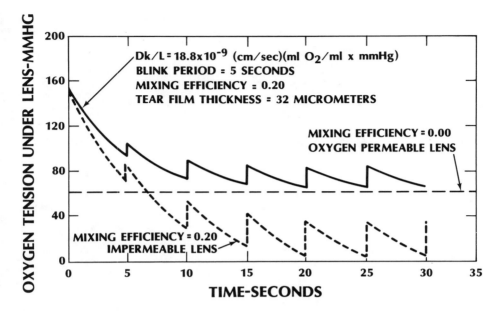

Figure 7.26 Oxygen tension under a rigid oxygen-permeable contact lens (RGP) when there is pumping (solid saw-tooth curve). The dashed saw-tooth curve is for an oxygen-impermeable contact lens (PMMA) that is pumping tear fluid under the lens with each blink. The horizontal dashed line gives the oxygen tension under the rigid gas-permeable lens when there is no tear pumping. (From Fatt I, Lin D [1976]: Oxygen tension under a contact lens during blinking—a comparison of theory and experimental observation. Am. J. Optom. 47:50–55.)

THE MULTILAYERED CORNEA

Mathematical methods for predicting oxygen tension within a hypothetical one-layer cornea or at the surface of the cornea have been examined up to this point. The more realistic multilayered cornea will now be examined. Although the mathematical methods needed for the multilayer cornea are beyond the scope of this text, they are similar in theory to the earlier discussion on the hypothetical one-layer cornea, and the results are important.

Figure 7.28 shows the oxygen tension inside a multilayered cornea as a function of the oxygen tension at the anterior surface. These curves were obtained by Fatt, Freeman, and Lin (1974) from data on rabbit corneal properties found by Freeman (1972) and Freeman and Fatt (1972) (see Table 7.2). Several interesting observations can be made.

First, oxygen tension in the endothelium is not significantly reduced even when the anterior surface oxygen tension approaches zero. The oxygen tension in the endothelium is set by that of the adjacent aqueous humor. This means that the metabolic dysfunction that results in corneal swelling when a tight-fitting oxygen-

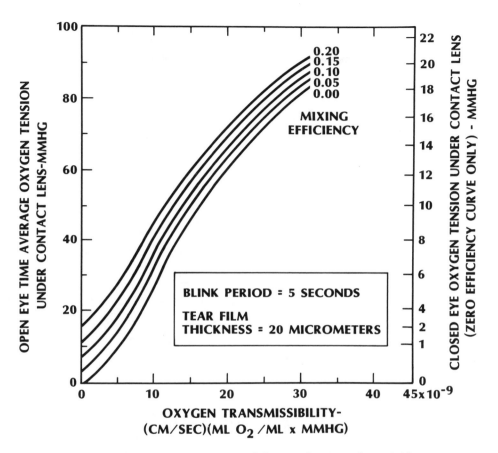

Figure 7.27 Time–average oxygen tension (*left vertical axis*) under a rigid gas-permeable contact lens (RGP) as a function of the oxygen transmissibility of the lens. Curves are for tear-mixing efficiencies (exchange with external tears) of from zero to 0.20. Blinking period is every 5 sec. A uniform tear layer of 20 μm under the lens is assumed. The right-hand vertical axis gives the oxygen tension under the lens in the closed eye and for the open eye when there is no tear exchange under the lens. (From Fatt and Liu, 1984).

impermeable contact lens is worn, or when a nitrogen goggle is used experimentally, cannot be associated with direct hypoxia at the endothelial side of the cornea.

Second, oxygen enters the cornea at *both* posterior and anterior surfaces because the slopes of all curves are seen to lead into the cornea.

Third, use of a tight, oxygen-impermeable contact lens or nitrogen goggle will make the epithelium totally anoxic. The epithelium cannot be supplied with oxygen from the aqueous humor because the endothelium and keratocytes of the

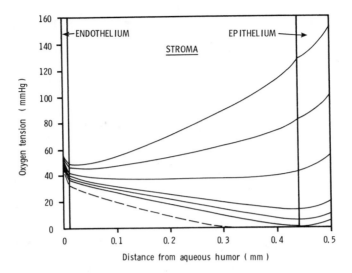

Figure 7.28 Oxygen tension profiles in the cornea for various oxygen tensions at the anterior surface. The upper curve represents the open eye; the third curve from the top is for the closed eye. The dashed curve is for an eye covered by an oxygen-impermeable tight contact lens or a nitrogen-filled goggle. All curves are intended to start at 55 mmHg on the left ordinate. (With permission from Fatt I, Freeman RD, Lin D [1974]: Exp. Eye Res. 18:357–365. Copyright by Academic Press Inc. [London] Ltd.)

stroma consume the oxygen diffusing from the posterior surface before it can reach the back of the epithelium. Weissman and associates (1981) calculated that the oxygen tension of the aqueous humor would need to increase to 200 mmHg or greater to enable oxygen to diffuse totally through the human cornea to the epithelium when the anterior corneal surface is made anoxic.

The method of calculation of Fatt, Freeman, and Lin (1974) can be extended to a four-layer cornea, where the fourth layer is an oxygen-permeable contact lens (tear exchange is disallowed in this model, and the lens is best considered a hydrogel as no tear layer is modeled between the lens and the cornea) by the method discussed above with the one-layer cornea. Figure 7.29 shows the oxygen tension profiles of a model three-layer cornea covered with a contact lens 0.1 mm thick under open-eye conditions (i.e., the oxygen tension of the anterior lens surface is set at 155 mmHg). The boundaries for the stroma–endothelium and stroma–epithelium are not drawn in, but these layers are modeled in the profiles and are indicated by the arrows at the bottom of the figure. Four different oxygen-permeable contact lens materials are modeled, indicated by *a, b, c,* and *d* on the profiles. Lenses made of materials *b* and *c* are predicted to be tolerated, as the oxygen tension under the lens for either is greater than 40 to 50 mmHg, but a lens made from material *d* would result in an oxygen tension of about 20 mmHg

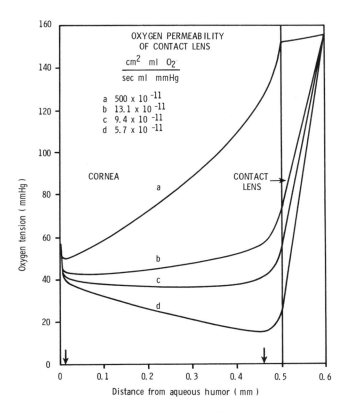

Figure 7.29 Oxygen tension profiles in the cornea of an *open eye* covered by an oxygen-permeable contact lens. Four profiles are shown to represent the effect of four different contact lens materials. All contact lenses are 0.1 mm thick. The arrows on the horizontal axis show the interface between (*left*) endothelium and stroma and (*right*) stroma and epithelium. (With permission from Fatt I, Freeman RD, Lin D [1974]: Exp. Eye Res. 18:357-265. Copyright by Academic Press Inc. [London] Ltd.)

at the anterior corneal surface, and some hypoxic effects would be predicted. Lens material *a* is so permeable it is practically "oxygen transparent."

Figure 7.30 is the same situation, but for the closed eye, where the anterior lens surface oxygen tension drops to 55 mmHg. Curves for materials *c* and *d* do not appear, since they do not allow oxygen to reach the epithelium under these conditions. A lens made of material *b* should also cause substantial metabolic changes as oxygen tension is predicted to be only about 2 mmHg. Material *a*, however, produces a lens that maintains oxygen tension at 50 mmHg even under closed-eye conditions; this is clearly a material to be sought, but this hypothetical material is not currently available.

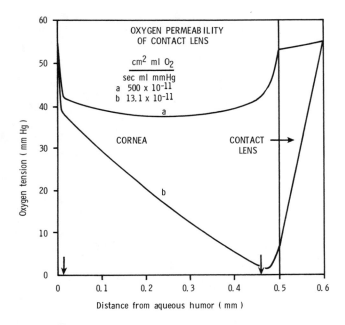

Figure 7.30 Oxygen tension profile in the cornea of a *closed eye* wearing an oxygen-permeable contact lens. Two profiles are shown to represent the effect of two different contact lens materials. The contact lenses are 0.1 mm thick. The arrows on the horizontal axis show the interface between (*left*) endothelium and stroma and (*right*) stroma and epithelium. (With permission from Fatt I, Freeman RD, Lin D [1974]: Exp. Eye Res. 18:357–365. Copyright by Academic Press Inc. [London] Ltd.)

CARBON DIOXIDE

The metabolism of glucose by the cornea leads to the production of both lactic acid and carbon dioxide. De Roetth (1950) found that the respiratory quotient was 1.00 in the ox cornea, which means that 1 mole of carbon dioxide is produced for every mole of oxygen consumed.

The movement of carbon dioxide (CO_2) in the cornea poses an interesting problem in contact lens application. The aqueous humor has substantial dissolved carbon dioxide; Fatt and Bieber (1968) originally suggested a carbon dioxide tension of 55 mmHg for the aqueous humor based on use of the Henderson-Hasselbalch relationship with the pH and bicarbonate content for the aqueous given by Davson (1962), but more recently Gamm (1980) found a slightly lower value of 40 mmHg. The atmosphere, however, has only a minute concentration of carbon dioxide; the carbon dioxide tension is about 0.3 mmHg. Therefore, the flux must be in the posterior-to-anterior direction across the cornea under open-eye conditions. In the absence of carbon dioxide production such situation would be profiled by a straight line across a model cornea with the aqueous humor boundary set at about 50 mmHg and the tear film at zero. Production of carbon dioxide in the tissues gives an upward bow to this line, perhaps arched more greatly in the areas of the endothelium and epithelium and more straight across the stroma—in response to the distribution of the cells that produce carbon dioxide.

The permeability of water to carbon dioxide is quite high, about 9×10^{-9} cm^2 ml CO$_2$/sec ml mmHg, which is 10 times the permeability of water to oxygen. In corneal tissues, Fatt and Bieber (1968) also felt that $D_e k_{CO_2}$ was high, about 20 times $D_e k_{O_2}$. This means that carbon dioxide coming from the aqueous humor and produced in the cornea can move easily toward the tears. Figure 7.31 shows a carbon dioxide profile in a model open-eye cornea—these calculations are similar to those described above for oxygen—assuming that the carbon dioxide tension in the aqueous humor is 55 mmHg and that all the oxygen utilized by the cornea is converted to carbon dioxide; note that this is the maximum possible situation, and the actual production rate may be less because much of the glucose consumed is converted to lactic acid and not completely reduced through aerobic glycolysis. Yet Figure 7.31 still shows an almost straight line, indicating that the metabolism of the cornea has little effect on the diffusion profile because the $D_e k_{CO_2}$ is so high.

The outward flux of carbon dioxide from the cornea of the open eye has been measured directly by Fatt, Hill, and Takahashi (1964) and found to be 21 μl CO$_2$/cm^2 hour. The product of the slope of the profile in Figure 7.31 times $D_e k_{CO_2}$ should give a similar term. If $D_e k_{O_2}$ for the cornea is taken from Table 7.2 and multiplied by 20 to get $D_e k_{CO_2}$, the CO$_2$ efflux is calculated to be about 10 μl CO$_2$/cm^2 hour, a very similar value considering the various approximations. These figures are higher than the respiratory quotient alone would suggest because of the efflux of carbon dioxide through the cornea from the aqueous humor, as shown in the model profiles discussed earlier.

When the eye is closed, the anterior surface of the cornea is exposed to the average carbon dioxide tension of the blood system in the palpebral conjunctiva, which is about 55 mmHg. In Figure 7.32, a dashed line shows the predicted carbon dioxide profile, considering the aqueous humor carbon dioxide tension to be 55 mmHg (which might be slightly high). It appears that carbon dioxide produced in the cornea diffuses equally toward both surfaces, and the profile is very flat at about 50 mmHg for these conditions.

A tight, carbon dioxide–impermeable contact lens will result in a similar profile, shown by the solid line in Figure 7.32. All the carbon dioxide produced in the cornea must diffuse posteriorly, as shown by the slope of this line. Consequently, there will be a slightly higher concentration of carbon dioxide in the cornea under the gas-impermeable contact lens than there is present in the cornea of the closed eye. The predicted increase in carbon dioxide tension at the anterior corneal surface is quite small, found here to be about 3 mmHg, and a similar value (about 10 mmHg) was experimentally found by Ang and Efron (1989). Ang and Efron (1989) also measured the Dk_{CO_2} of contact lens materials and found that there was about a 20-fold increase in Dk_{CO_2} (compared to Dk_{O_2}) for hydrogels

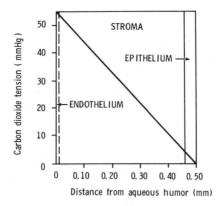

Figure 7.31 Carbon dioxide tension profile in the cornea of an open eye. (With permission from Fatt I [1968]: Exp. Eye Res. 7: 413–430. Copyright by Academic Press Inc. [London] Ltd.)

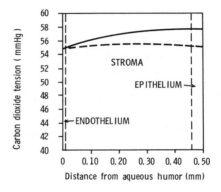

Figure 7.32 Carbon dioxide tension profile in the cornea of a closed eye (----); and profile in a cornea covered by a tight, impermeable contact lens (—). (With permission from Fatt I [1968]: Exp. Eye Res. 7:413–430. Copyright by Academic Press Inc. [London] Ltd.)

and about a 6-fold increase for rigid gas-permeable materials; the latter figure was confirmed by Fatt and Fink (1989). Use of a carbon dioxide–permeable contact lens under open-eye conditions will decrease the CO_2 tension under the lens, whereas under closed-eye conditions the CO_2 tension should be relatively flat across the system, as predicted in Figure 7.32. Such values could be calculated in a manner similar to that discussed above for oxygen but have been measured experimentally by Ang and Efron (1989). They found values ranging between 5 and 40 mmHg, dependent on Dk/L_{CO_2}, for the open eye, and about 40 ± 5 mmHg for the closed eye, as expected.

Do these changes in carbon dioxide during contact lens wear have any effect on the cornea? Some clinicians have attributed a "burning" sensation, occasionally described by contact lens—wearing patients, to a change in the pH in the tears under the lens caused by accumulation of CO_2. A 3-mmHg increase in CO_2 tension is too low, however, to have much effect; it should only decrease the pH by about 0.01. Recent studies, however, suggest that these CO_2 changes may cause more problems when they are inside the cornea. Bonanno and Polse (1987) found that raising the CO_2 tension at the anterior corneal surface to about 40 mmHg (by use of humidified gas in a goggle experiment or with wear of a contact lens) decreased stromal pH from 7.53 to 7.16 (mean values from six subjects). Others (Holden et al. 1985) have hypothesized that such a pH change in the stroma may affect both endothelial morphology and function.

CORNEAL THICKNESS CONTROL

The normal cornea maintains a relatively constant thickness in the face of an ever-present imbibition pressure in the stroma (see Chapter 6) that acts to draw water continuously across the limiting cellular layers. As shown in Chapter 6, the optical properties of the cornea are dependent on the maintenance of an appropriate thickness; a swollen stroma scatters light and reduces visual acuity.

To explain the maintenance of corneal thickness, early students of corneal physiology believed that the limiting layers of the cornea, the endothelium and epithelium, were so impermeable to water that they formed absolute barriers to water imbibition by the stroma. These layers are now known to be permeable to water, as we discussed in Chapter 6, and over a longer or shorter time the stroma should draw water across them.

A second hypothesis to explain the observed constancy of corneal thickness invoked an osmotic pressure difference between the stromal fluid and the outer fluids: the tears and aqueous humor. The stromal fluid was proposed to be lower in concentration than the outside fluids so that osmosis would transfer excess fluid from inside the cornea to outside. There are several objections to this hypothesis. First, the limiting layers would have to be *absolutely* impermeable to whatever dissolved species is setting up the osmotic pressure difference between the inside and outside of the stroma. If either layer is even slightly permeable to this species, diffusion will eventually equalize the concentration difference and the osmotic driving force disappears. Second, if the stroma swells, for whatever reason, the passive osmotic pressure model has no mechanism for ejecting the dissolved species that must have entered the stroma to cause the swelling.

These two objections led physiologists to seek a corneal-thickness control mechanism that operates through the metabolic work of the corneal cells. It was easy to show that this control had to be in the limiting layers; if the epithelium and endothelium are scraped off the cornea of a living eye, the stroma swells and cannot return to its usual thickness. That this control was through cellular metabolism was shown elegantly by Davson (1955) in his well-known "temperature-reversal" experiment. Davson placed the enucleated eye of a rabbit in a moist, air-filled chamber and noted that the cornea maintained its thickness for several hours at 37°C. When the temperature was reduced to 10°C for several hours, however, the cornea swelled. If the eye was returned to 37°C, the cornea would return to almost its normal thickness, but this return could be prevented either by withholding oxygen from the cornea during the warming or by applying metabolic inhibitors to the cornea. Others subsequently showed that glucose was consumed in the temperature-reversal phenomenon. Since this effect only occurs with the epithelium and endothelium in place, it must be located in one (or both) of these layers. But which layer?

Some researchers found evidence that the epithelium transports sodium ion from the tears into the stroma, thereby generating a transepithelial potential of about 30 mV (in the rabbit), and suggested this could reduce the swelling power of the stroma. Fatt (1968a), however, showed that the stroma can still swell in salt concentrations as high as 10% and found no experimental evidence that stromal fluid is more than 1% salt concentration (see Figure 6.8). Subsequent studies have confirmed an active absorption of sodium ion but have observed that this is balanced by an outward chlorine ion secretion (that can be neurophysiologically or chemically modulated), which results in a zero net solute transfer in the presence of the resting potential and without pharmacological intervention (Klyce and Crosson 1985).

Maurice (1972) carried out an elegant experiment to demonstrate that the endothelium alone, although not the source of much of the resting potential in the cornea, can pump water against an opposing resistance. Figure 7.33 shows his data, with the apparatus shown in the upper left-hand corner. A section of stroma with an intact endothelial layer was clamped between water-filled chambers. The outlet tube from the left-hand chamber, the endothelial side of the tissue specimen, was higher than the tube connected to the right-hand chamber. At 35°C, water moved into the upper tube and out of the lower tube. This movement required work against the gravitational head of water in the tubes. Quickly changing the temperature of the apparatus to 0°C stopped all water movement in the tubes. When returned to 35°C (right-hand side of the graph), the water movement resumed. Note that the slopes of the curves for 35°C are the same, both before and after the cooling interruption (at a thinning rate of some 60 μm/hour). This means that true water movement was observed that was not an artifact induced by swelling of the tissue or expansion of water within the equipment. The observation that this process stopped when the tissue was cooled and started again when it was warmed makes it likely that this is associated with the previously discussed temperature-reversal effect. In addition, the thinning rate observed by Maurice is similar to the swelling rate noted earlier by Trenberth and Mishima (1968a, b) (45 μm/hour) when they poisoned the active transport mechanism with ouabain without affecting endothelial permeability.

Most corneal biophysicists have embraced Maurice's work and accept that the endothelium is responsible for maintaining corneal hydration and secondarily transparency. But what does the endothelium pump? It is unlikely that water itself is actively transported. Hodson and Miller (1976) found that the endothelial cells

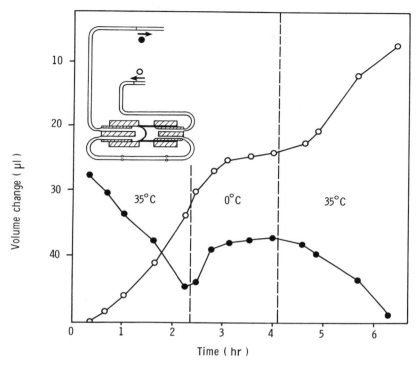

Figure 7.33   Transfer of liquid from the lower outlet tube ○, to the upper outlet tube ●, in the double-chamber system when inlet tubes are kept closed. The tissue was a fresh cornea with epithelium and most of the stroma excised away. The liquid medium was gassed with 95% O_2, 5% CO_2. Temperature of the water bath was as indicated on graph. (From Maurice DM [1972]: The location of the fluid pump in the cornea. J. Physiol. 221:43–54.)

actively transport bicarbonate ions into the anterior chamber, and water tends to follow osmotically. Two-thirds of the substrate is provided by bicarbonate ions originating in the stroma, and the remainder is provided by the intracellular conversion of exogenous carbon dioxide into bicarbonate.

But if the endothelium is responsible for maintaining corneal thickness (hydration and transparency) by pumping bicarbonate into the anterior chamber, and if it receives all of its metabolic needs such as glucose, amino acids, and oxygen from the immediately adjacent aqueous humor, and as this source is not theoretically interrupted by events on the anterior surface as we modeled above, why is it that the cornea swells when a contact lens (or nitrogen goggle) reduces *external* oxygen supply?

One possibility might be that anterior anoxia depresses epithelial metabolism and then this layer becomes more mechanically leaky to water: that is, its hydraulic conductivity increases when its metabolism is interrupted. We know from the early work of Smelser and Ozanics (1952) and Uniacke and co-workers (1972) that epithelial glycogen stores disappear under conditions of epithelial hypoxia. Wilson, Fatt, and Freeman (1973), however, showed that the water permeability of this layer is unchanged when it is made anoxic. They also showed that, although the epithelium itself may not be affected by anoxia, it may play some role in the swelling process under these conditions. Figure 7.34 shows the thickness of a rabbit stroma when a 1% saline solution bathing the epithelium is switched from aerated to deaerated. (The microscope through which this observation was made could distinguish stromal thickness from epithelial thickness.) There was little change in epithelial layer thickness (3%), but the stroma swelled 20%.

The data of Wilson, Fatt, and Freeman (1973) also showed that the swelling of the stroma began within 10 minutes of making the epithelium anoxic. The time needed for a soluble substance to diffuse from the epithelium to the endothelium can be calculated from

$$t = \frac{L^2}{D_e} \tag{7.86}$$

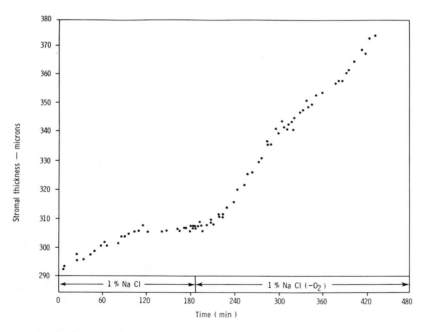

Figure 7.34 Swelling of the stroma when the epithelial surface is made anoxic by bathing with a deaerated 1% NaCl solution. During the first 180 minutes after mounting the preparation, the epithelium was bathed with aerated 1% NaCl solution. The endothelial surface is covered with silicone oil. The swelling rate of the stroma during anoxia is 21.8 μm/hour during the first hour. (With permission from Wilson GS, Fatt I, Freeman RD [1973]: Exp. Eye Res. 17:165. Copyright by Academic Press Inc. [London] Ltd.)

where L is the distance between the epithelium and endothelium and D_e is the diffusion coefficient of the diffusing species. If t is 640 seconds (about 11 minutes) and L is 0.4 mm (for rabbit stroma), then D_e is 0.25×10^{-5} cm^2/sec; this is about 0.1 of that of oxygen in stroma, and approximately that predicted for a large molecule. Wilson, Fatt, and Freeman (1973) concluded that this time course suggests that the anoxic epithelium might produce some large molecule that crosses the stroma to cause a reduction in the pumping work by the endothelial cells.

Klyce (1981) considered this observation and then experimentally determined that increased production of *lactate ions* by hypoxic epithelial cells could provide the large molecule that diffuses across the stroma. His data indicate that excess lactate diffuses across the stroma to act osmotically to counterbalance the effect of the pumped bicarbonate ions from the stroma to the aqueous humor.

The above discussion indicates that the cornea is in a steady state of dehydration that maintains the spacing of the stromal collagen fibers to promote transparency. A force generated by stromal swelling pressure acts in the direction that would result in water being drawn into the cornea, but this is counterbalanced by the active transport of an osmotically active ion, probably bicarbonate, from the stroma to the anterior chamber by the endothelial cells. When the corneal surface oxygen tension drops below the level needed for aerobic metabolism, excess lactate is produced by the hypoxic epithelial cells. Lactate cannot diffuse between the tight borders of the epithelial cells and therefore moves backward to the endothelium where it can partially counteract the effect of the bicarbonate ion, resulting in stromal swelling. Mechanical or chemical insults may also affect the barrier role of either limiting layer, or directly or indirectly the endothelial pump, to result in corneal swelling.

Clinical studies have shown that corneal thickness is also affected by the salt content of the tear film. The salt content of the tear film is about 10% greater in the open eye than that of freshly produced tears owing to evaporation of water from the relatively warm (35°C) tears. When the eye is closed, during sleep, for example, evaporation is reduced and the cornea is bathed in fresh tears. Mandell and Fatt (1965) found that there is an approximately 5% increase in corneal thickness during sleep. It was originally believed that the cornea was acting as an osmometer in this situation, in which the epithelium is the semipermeable membrane; the lower salt content of fresh tears under the closed eyelid should cause the stroma to imbibe water across the epithelium by osmosis.

Because of the changing definition of the "critical oxygen tension," however, some now believe that the normal upper lid may not supply enough oxygen to the anterior corneal surface to totally prevent metabolic swelling under closed-eye conditions, and hence perhaps part of the small (5%) "physiological" swelling observed during sleep is due to the osmotic changes in the tears and another part may be due to hypoxia through the mechanism described above.

Although stromal swelling occurs when a hypotonic solution is applied to the eye, it must be recalled that the epithelial cells may also swell. The epithelial cells are not unlike other cells, such as red blood cells, in this respect. Wilson and

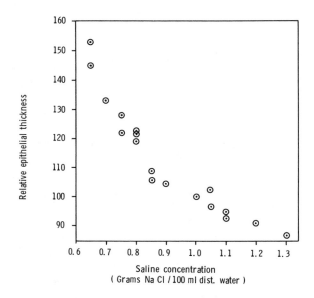

Figure 7.35 Thickness of the epithelium in an excised but living cornea as a function of the NaCl concentration of the solution bathing the anterior surface. (From Wilson GS, Fatt I [1974]: Thickness changes in the epithelium of the excised rabbit cornea. Am. J. Optom. 51:75–83.)

Fatt (1974) have shown that epithelial thickness is directly related to saline concentration of a bathing fluid. Figure 7.35 shows epithelial thickness as a function of solution concentration, with the thickness in 1% NaCl taken as a value of 100.

If the normal open eye has a tear film that is concentrated by evaporation to 1.1% NaCl and the closed eye is exposed to isotonic tears (equivalent to 1.0% NaCl), Figure 7.35 shows there should be a 5% swelling of the epithelium under the closed eyelid. Since the human epithelium is about 50 μm thick, this would mean the epithelium should thicken about 2.5 μm. Mandell and Fatt (1965), however, observed a 5% increase in total corneal thickness, amounting to some 20 to 25 μm. Thus, hypotonic solutions on the eye can thicken both epithelium and stroma, but in the range observed in the human eye most of the observed change is stromal.

Mandell and Harris (1968) presented an interesting study of corneal swelling due to fresh tears. They measured 3% corneal swelling in one eye when a rigid contact lens was worn on the *other* eye. Clearly such thickening could not be related to oxygen deprivation. Instead, it is clear that bilateral lacrimation caused by the contact lens on one eye bathed the lens-free cornea with fresh tears, a solution less concentrated than that normally present. The cornea responded to this less than normally concentrated solution by swelling, acting just as an osmometer. This process obviously occurs under such conditions at a rate greater than the endothelium can remove this excess water from the stroma.

8

The Sclera

The sclera is a thin spherically shaped connective tissue contiguous with the cornea at the limbus. The stromal lamellae from the cornea, on crossing through the limbus, increasingly interweave (Figure 8.1). Individual collagen fibrils of each lamella also change from their uniform 30-nm diameter and 60-nm center-to-center spacing in the cornea to a wide variety of diameters (30 to 300 nm) and irregular spacing in the sclera.

The water content of the sclera is about 70% compared to the 78% of the corneal stroma. Of the solid material in the sclera, Hogan and co-workers (1971) suggest that 75% is collagen, 10% other proteins, 1% glycosaminoglycans (GAGs) (note, for comparison, that the corneal stroma is 4.5% GAGs), and the rest salt. This composition appears to be based on an early gravimetric analysis of bovine sclera; when a modern biochemical selective digestion procedure was used, about 50% of the solid matter of human sclera, by weight, was found to be collagen, predominantly type I (Keeley et al. 1984).

Nerves and blood vessels pierce the sclera, but in the living eye the blood vessels are filled and under internal pressure, and therefore fit tightly into their passages through the sclera. There are few blood vessels traveling laterally in the sclera; the blood vessels seen grossly on the "white" of the eye are traveling within the loose episcleral tissue, which lies on top of the sclera itself. These vessels are densely packed near the corneal margin. The inner surface of the sclera is covered with the highly vascular choroid.

The sclera contains cells similar to those found in the corneal stroma (fibroblasts) and, in addition, large numbers of pigmented cells (melanocytes and pigmented macrophages), particularly on its inner surface. The noncellular lamellae lie parallel to the limbus in the anterior portion of the sclera and run on the meridian at the equator, that is, roughly anterior to posterior. Lamellae begin to cross each other as they travel more posteriorly until, at the posterior pole of the eye, they are traveling circularly around the exit of the optic nerve—except for some bundles of scleral collagen that extend across the approximately 2- to 3-mm diameter opening to form the meshwork of the *lamina cribrosa* (Hogan et al. 1971). The collagen bundles vary considerably in size and and shape, and they

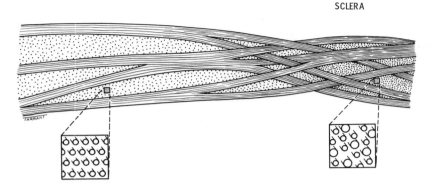

Figure 8.1 Diagrammatic representation of the cornea and sclera showing the difference in structure of the two tissues. (From Davson H [ed] [1969]: The Eye, Vol. 1. New York, Academic Press.)

branch extensively, intermingling in various planes. Friberg and Lace (1988) found that the modulus of elasticity for strips of human sclera varied with location and stiffened with age of the individual, averaging 2.9 ($\pm$ 1.4) $\times$ $10^6 N/m^2$ for anterior sclera and 1.8 ($\pm$ 1.1) $\times$ $10^6 N/m^2$ for posterior sclera at stress levels ranging from 20 to 260 $\times$ $10^4 N/m^2$. They referenced an earlier author's explanation of this difference to the more uniform weave and orientation of anterior collagen lamellae compared to a looser weave in the posterior lamellae.

The thickness of the sclera varies from 0.6 mm at the limbus down to 0.5 mm at the equator and then up to 1 mm or more at the exit of the optic nerve. It is not clear how the sclera changes in thickness from point to point. If the lamellae are continuous and of the same dry thickness at all points, extra-thick areas must contain larger amounts of water. On the other hand, extra-thick areas may be composed of more layers of lamellae. The thickness–hydration relationships of human and rabbit sclera are shown in Figure 8.2.

SWELLING PRESSURE, DIFFUSION, AND BULK FLOW

The swelling pressure versus hydration curve of the sclera is very different from that of the stroma (Figure 8.3). This difference is attributable to the lower GAG content of the sclera. The hydration of the sclera is about 2 gm water/gm dry material near the limbus, and the corresponding swelling pressure is 10 to 17 mmHg (14 to 23 gm/cm^2). In the adjacent corneal stroma the hydration is 3.5 gm water/gm dry material, and the swelling pressure has increased to 60 mmHg. From physical principles, it can be said that a difference in steady-state swelling pressure in adjacent tissues can exist only if there is a flow of water from one to

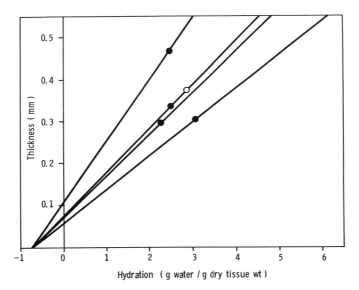

Figure 8.2 Thickness as a function of hydration for rabbit sclera (●) and human sclera
(○). (With permission from Fatt I, Hedbys BO [1970]: Flow of water in the sclera. Exp.
Eye Res. 19:243 Copyright by Academic Press Inc. [London] Ltd.)

the other. Since the corneal stroma has the higher swelling pressure (corresponding to a greater negative pressure), water will flow from the sclera into the cornea.
Maurice (1969) and Fatt and Hedbys (1970b) have calculated this flow rate to be
0.15 μl/hour. This represents only about 3% of the water being kept out of the
stroma by the endothelial pump (as estimated by Maurice [1969]) and therefore
should not be a serious extra load on the dehydrating mechanism of the cornea.
Additional data supporting the existence of such a flow of water have recently
been provided by Wiig (1989, 1990).

A postulated flow of water from the sclera to the cornea poses a problem,
however, when one attempts to explain the extra thickness of the stroma at the
limbus. It was earlier suggested that the limbal region of the corneal stroma was
thicker because either there was more dry material of constant hydration or
constant dry material of increased hydration at this site (see Chapter 6). If there
is a flow of water from the sclera to the corneal stroma, it might seem reasonable
that water will continue to flow radially some distance into the cornea before
being removed. If this is indeed the steady-state condition, then the stromal limbus
could be thicker because it is at a higher hydration and lower swelling pressure.

Maurice and Polgar (1977) measured the diffusion of several chemicals in
beef sclera in an effort to arrive at a description of the passage of ophthalmic
pharmaceutical agents. They found that the sclera was impermeable to most dyes
studied, except for two negatively charged and relatively small (by molecular
weight) chemicals: fluorescein and acid fuchsin. A variety of ions and solutes up

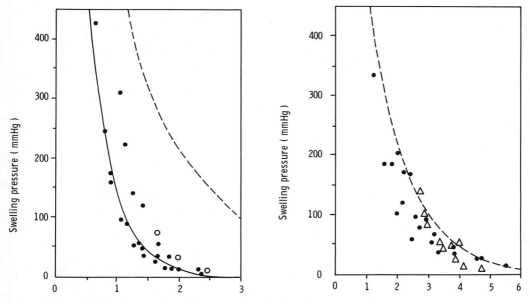

Figure 8.3 *Left,* swelling pressure as a function of hydration for rabbit (●) and human sclera (○). ——, least squares straight line fitted to rabbit sclera data plotted as logarithm of swelling pressure versus hydration; ----, rabbit stroma. *Right,* swelling pressure as a function of hydration for human stroma at 25°C. ●, data from Fatt and Hedbys (1970a); Δ, data from Hedbys and Dohlman (1963). ----, least squares line fitted to rabbit stroma data plotted as logarithm of swelling pressure versus hydration. (With permission from Fatt I, Hedbys BO [1970]: Flow of water in the sclera. Exp. Eye Res. 10:243. Copyright by Academic Press Inc. [London] Ltd.)

to the size of serum albumin were found to diffuse about three times more slowly in beef sclera than in rabbit corneal stroma, with diffusion being in inverse relationship to molecular weight, as expected.

The flow conductivity of the sclera has been found to be considerably greater than that of the corneal stroma at all hydrations (Figure 8.4); this is attributable to the lower GAG content of the sclera. The measured flow conductivity of the sclera can be used to calculate the outflow of aqueous humor from the eye via the sclera. This calculation can ignore the flow resistance of the retina because Fatt and Shantinath (1971) have shown that retinal resistance is insignificant compared to that of the sclera. The resistances of the vitreous body, choroid, and pigment epithelium are likewise assumed to be unimportant when compared to that of the sclera.

Darcy's law for flow conductivity is given by Equation 6.13. For human sclera, the flow conductivity (k/μ) is about 15×10^{-13} cm^4 dynes^{-1} sec^{-1}, as measured by Fatt and Hedbys (1970b) at room temperature (25°C).* The area of

*To obtain k/μ for the sclera at ocular temperature (37°C), the value of k/μ at 25°C is multiplied by μ_{25}/μ_{37}, which is 1.29, and k/μ at 37°C is found to be 19.3×10^{-13} cm^4 dynes^{-1} sec^{-1} (see Table 9.1).

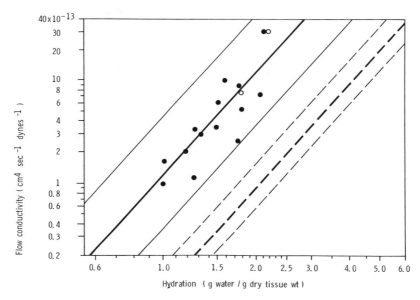

Figure 8.4 Flow conductivity as a function of hydration for rabbit sclera (●) and human sclera (○). ——, fitted by the method of least squares to the sclera data. ----, the best fitted line through rabbit stroma data points (not shown). The outer lines represent the 95% confidence limits. (With permission from Fatt I, Hedbys BO [1970]: Flow of water in the sclera. Exp. Eye Res. 10:243. Copyright by Academic Press Inc. [London] Ltd.)

the sclera in humans is 11.5 cm^2, and its average thickness can be taken as 0.06 cm. An intraocular pressure of about 17 mmHg is taken as the driving force because the pressure in the loose episcleral tissue on the outer surface of the sclera is not likely to be above atmospheric pressure. The flow rate calculated from Equation 6.13 is then 0.53 μl/min. This is about 21% of the total outflow of aqueous humor (estimated at 2.5 μl/min), in agreement with the experimental results of Kleinstein and Fatt (1977).

TISSUE MECHANICS OF SCLERA (AND CORNEA)

The elastic properties of the sclera have been discussed in Chapter 3, where the concept of ocular rigidity was considered. The corneal stroma and sclera provide the strength of the tough outer tunic of the eye. This strength allows the eye to be an inflated spheroid that is very resistant to external impact. The soft cellular linings of both cornea and sclera (the episclera outside, and choroid and retina inside, in the latter case) have little or no mechanical strength themselves.

The sclera forms 93% of the area of the human eye, and therefore any extension of the eye when pressure is increased is primarily a result of scleral stretching.

The internal pressure of the eye (intraocular pressure, or IOP) is the source of tension in the sclera and corneal stroma. Tension has the dimensions of force per unit length and can be related to the internal pressure of a perfect sphere as follows: a fluid under pressure in a sphere must apply a force normal to the surface of the shell at all points, because, by definition, fluids do not support shearing stresses. This stress pattern is shown in Figure 8.5. Each normal force has a component that projects down to a disk formed by a plane passing through the equator of the sphere. As a result, the two hemispheres are each experiencing a force (F) (equal to the internal pressure multiplied by the area projected onto the plane through the equator) that is tending to separate them:

$$F = \text{IOP}\pi R^2 \tag{8.1}$$

where R is the radius of the circle. The length of any equatorial circle on the surface of the sphere is simply the circumference of the sphere: $2\pi R$. Therefore, the tension force per unit length is

$$T = \text{IOP} \frac{\pi R^2}{2 \pi R} = \text{IOP} \frac{R}{2} \tag{8.2}$$

Since the cornea has a smaller radius of curvature than does the sclera, Equation 8.2 predicts a smaller tension in the cornea.

This stress situation becomes more complex at the limbus where there is a discontinuity in the curvature of the globe. The tangential tension in the sclera (T_s) is not matched at the limbus by an equal tangential tension in the corneal stroma (T_c), but yet there is a stationary equilibrium; therefore there must be another force (called T_L in Figure 8.6) opposing them. Maurice (1969) has compared T_L to the force applied by a purse string drawn around a perfect sphere, forming the indentation at the limbus called the *corneal sulcus*. T_L is greater than either T_s or

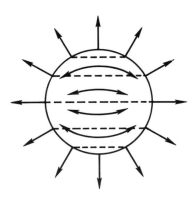

Figure 8.5 Stress pattern in the shell of an inflated sphere.

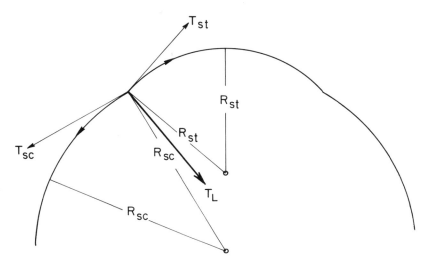

Figure 8.6 Stress vector pattern at the limbus. T_{sc} *and* T_s are the sclera and stroma, respectively, at the junction between these two tissues.

T_c, and the limbal region supports this extra tension by being thicker (and perhaps richer in circular collagen fibers) than either the central cornea or equatorial sclera.

The sclera is reported to have an elastic modulus in circumferential tension from 10^7 to 10^9 dynes/cm^2, with a tendency for the sclera to become less compliant (higher modulus) as the applied stress increases. This can be attributed to the tendency of collagen fibrils to be wavy at low levels of stress but to become increasingly taut as the applied stress increases. Battaglioli and Kamm (1984) found that the elastic modulus for circumferential compressive stress was 10^2 greater than for radial compressive stress, consistent with the concept that the collagen fibrils run in the circumferential direction. When a radial compressive stress is applied, the bundles of collagen fibers are compacted; this process requires far less stress than stretching these fibers.

9

Retina

The retina is a highly complex nervous tissue that converts light energy first to chemical energy and then to electrical energy to process visual information. The retina is actually an extension of the forebrain of the central nervous system. Our ability to observe the form and function of the retina, both for its own sake and as representative of the brain, has led to much interesting research.

To carry out its function as a transducer and processor of visual information, the retina must be structurally and biochemically maintained against the forces that tend to degrade it. These mechanisms are the major topics of this chapter. Photochemical changes that occur in the retinal pigments will also be described, but no attempt will be made here to link photochemistry to the visual process as this is beyond the scope of vegetative physiology.

STRUCTURE

The retina is a thin and delicate tissue lining the inner aspect of the eye. Grossly, the retina consists of a central portion at the posterior pole, about 5 to 6 mm in diameter, containing the concentric macula and fovea (the site of most acute vision). The peripheral retina extends anteriorly to the ora serrata. The retina varies in thickness from about 0.5 to 0.1 mm, being thickest around the optic disk and thinning at the ora serrata, the equator, and the fovea (Hogan et al. 1971).

The retina is customarily subdivided into ten layers easily identified with stains and the light microscope. These are (in order, from outside inward) (1) retinal pigment epithelium (RPE), (2) photoreceptor layer, (3) outer limiting membrane, (4) outer nuclear layer, (5) outer plexiform layer, (6) inner nuclear layer, (7) inner plexiform layer, (8) ganglion cell layer, (9) nerve fiber layer, and (10) inner limiting membrane. The innermost nine layers (excluding the RPE) are considered the *neural retina*.

The *rods* and *cones* are the sensory photoreceptor cells (approximately 100 million and 6 to 7 million per human retina, respectively), and their outer segments contain photosensitive pigments that initiate excitatory responses to light.

The external surfaces of the pigment epithelium cells lie flat against *Bruch's membrane* of the choroid, but the apical (inner) sides of these cells are characterized by numerous microvillous processes that cross an extracellular or *"subretinal"* space to interdigitate with and in some cases ensheath the outer segments of the photoreceptors. This intimate relationship is also physiological because the pigment epithelium consumes disks of the outer segments as they are shed by the photoreceptors to continue the functionally necessary constant renewal of these cells (first described by Young [1967]). The cell bodies (inner segments) of the rods and cones form the outer nuclear layer. The photoreceptors join bipolar and horizontal cells. The bipolar cells in turn connect to amacrine cells. These three cell types form the middle retinal layers. Visual processing begins with these complex interconnections. Ganglion cells then carry visual information along through the nerve fiber layer to the rest of the central nervous system (Hogan et al. 1971; Michels et al. 1990).

The glial cells (Müller cells) extend the full thickness of the retina; their expanded "feet" produce the vitreal face of the retina, composing much of the internal limiting membrane, while they separate the individual photoreceptors one from another on the outer surface. Within the retina, Müller cell processes fill in almost all the volume not occupied by other cells (e.g., nerves and rare astrocytes) and blood vessels, providing metabolic support to the nerve cells. There may be no physical barrier limiting diffusion within the retina (Cohen 1975).

METABOLISM

The retina receives its nutrition (e.g., glucose, oxygen, and importantly vitamin A or *retinol*) primarily from the retinal and choroidal blood circulatory systems. The retina will cease function in about 80 minutes if its blood supply is eliminated. (A small amount of nutrient material may be supplied from the vitreous as well; see Chapter 4.) There are two distinct blood supplies. The inner retina is supplied by the retinal vasculature (two capillary beds, one in the nerve fiber layer and the other in the inner nuclear layer), but the outer layers receive their nutrients by diffusion through Bruch's membrane from the choriocapillaris of the choroid. Thus there should be a physiological "watershed" area somewhere in the middle retina.

Retinal tissue has a high rate of oxygen consumption. Cohen and Noell (1965) measured rabbit oxygen uptake at 18 μl/mg dry weight hour (for comparison, Freeman [1972] found rabbit corneal endothelium oxygen uptake to be about 16 μl/mg dry weight hour). Zuckerman and Weiter (1980) found that the bullfrog retina consumes about 2.57×10^{-3} ml O_2/ml sec (compared to rabbit corneal endothelial consumption discussed above [see Table 7.2] at 1.4×10^{-3} ml O_2/ml sec); these authors suggested that most oxygen is consumed at the level of the photoreceptor inner segments, this consumption being necessary to maintain a high level of metabolism that includes active transport processes.

Studies report that the oxygen tension of the immediately preretinal vitreous in several mammalian species is about 10 to 30 mmHg while the animals breathe room air but increases to perhaps 50 to 100 mmHg under conditions of hyperoxia. Oxygen tension in the immediately preretinal vitreous is also heterogeneously distributed with regard to retinal vasculature, that is, higher over arteries and lower over veins (Linsenmeier et al. 1981; Linsenmeier and Yancey 1989; Pournaras et al. 1989; Yu et al. 1990).

Adler and co-workers (1983), working with cats, showed that the preretinal oxygen tension was quite similar to that found just within the retina, but oxygen tension profiles suggested that this value decreases somewhere near the inner segments of the photoreceptors and then rises again toward the choroidal face of the tissue. Because these authors found a steep rise in oxygen tension toward Bruch's membrane, in parallel to a rise in its electrical resistance, they suggested that this layer has a lower $D_e k$ (for oxygen) than that of the tissues on either side.

Oxygen tension in the retinas of several mammalian species (i.e., rabbits, cats, and rhesus monkeys) has been shown to *decrease* under conditions of darkness and *increase* with illumination, suggesting that retinal oxygen consumption decreases with light and increases in the dark (Stefansson et al. 1983; Tillis et al. 1988; Linsenmeier and Yancey 1989).

Increasing intraocular pressure (IOP) also appears to affect retinal oxygenation. Yancey and Linsenmeier (1989) found that the oxygen tension in the inner retina of cats was minimally affected but that the outer retina (supplied by the choroidal circulation) suffered a depression in oxygen tension of about 0.5 mmHg/mmHg increase in IOP. A reduction in oxygen supply to the retina brought on by an increase in IOP could adversely affect the physiology of the photoreceptor layer.

Finally, panretinal photocoagulation has been shown to raise preretinal oxygen tension over treated areas, corresponding to areas of loss of the mitochondria-rich photoreceptor inner segments (Molnar et al. 1985; Novack et al. 1990). This suggests that destruction of the oxygen-consuming photoreceptors results in an overall increase in oxygen supply to the inner retina.

According to Graymore (1969), Warburg studied a great many tissues and noted that the retina had the highest rate of anaerobic and aerobic glycolysis and respiration of any tissue he had examined. Despite this high rate of respiration, however, the oxidation of pyruvate in the mitochondria (principally in ellipsoid regions of the photoreceptor outer segments) does not keep pace with pyruvate production from glucose. Unusually, excess pyruvate is converted to lactic acid even though there is sufficient oxygen. There is some evidence that retinal cells can use this lactic acid as a fuel for further production of energy; the only other tissues that have such an ability are muscles and the liver. There is probably some degree of pentose phosphate activity in the mature retina as well. Glycogen is stored in the Müller cells (Kuwabara and Cogan 1961), which also have glycolytic enzymes such as lactic acid dehydrogenase. The retinal cells are also unique in that they are able to incorporate CO_2 into larger organic molecules, a process termed *carbon dioxide fixation* (Figure 9.1).

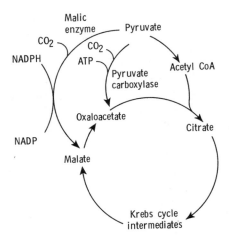

Figure 9.1 Possible routes for fixation of carbon dioxide via the pyruvate carboxylase or malic enzyme systems.

PHOTOCHEMISTRY

Light is effective in stimulating the retina because it is absorbed in the outer segments of photoreceptors. Substances that have the property of absorbing in that portion of the electromagnetic spectrum known as light are called *pigments*. If a substance absorbs all wavelengths of light equally, it appears gray or black. A red pigment, however, absorbs light of all wavelengths except red (Figure 9.2). Most of the pigments in the visual cells are not limited in their absorption to one small band of wavelengths but rather absorb, to a greater or lesser extent, over a broad range of the spectrum. The peak of each pigment's absorption curve is called its *absorption maximum*.

An example of a visual pigment is *rhodopsin,* which is found in the disks of the rod outer segments and has the absorption spectrum shown in Figure 9.3. Similar visual pigments are found in the cones. Rhodopsin has been intensively studied. It absorbs primarily yellow wavelengths of light, transmitting violet and red to appear purple by transmitted light; it is therefore called *visual purple.* Rhodopsin is a protein that is insoluble in water but can be taken into solution if detergent is added. It is sensitive to heat and chemical agents (acetone, ethanol, strong acids or alkalis) that denature protein. Its molecular weight is about 40,000.

Rhodopsin consists of a protein called *opsin* and a carotinoid called *retinal* (the aldehyde of vitamin A). Photons are absorbed by rhodopsin and induce a change in shape of retinal from its 11-*cis* to its all-*trans* forms (Figure 9.4). These are isomers; that is, the chemical "backbone" of this molecule changes shape but

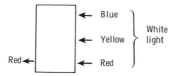

Figure 9.2 The mechanism by which a pigment appears red. All wave-lengths in white light except the red are absorbed.

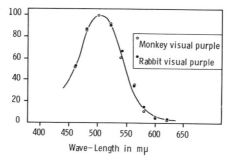

Figure 9.3 The absorption spectrum of rhodopsin of rabbit and monkey. Wavelength is in nm. The vertical axis represents absorption relative to that at 500.

there is no change in composition. This particular change in shape occurs by rotation between the carbon positions as shown in Figure 9.5.

The process by which retinal changes its shape facilitates binding of rhodopsin to a protein known as transducin. This binding alters the conformation of transducin, which in turn begins a cascade of biochemical reactions that lead to a change in the concentration of cyclic GMP* within the photoreceptor. The change in cyclic GMP is directly responsible for producing the electrical response that signals photoexcitation. Recent experiments indicate that calcium also plays an important role in the response of the receptors, probably by serving as an internal messenger for sensitivity modulation (light adaptation; see Fain and Mathews 1990). Used retinoids leave the photoreceptors, cross the subretinal space, and are stored in the RPE, where all-*trans* retinal is re-isomerized to 11-*cis* retinal. Eventually some retinal is recycled by being returned to the photoreceptors.

In the retina of a living animal, under constant light stimulation, a steady state must exist under which the rate at which the photochemicals are bleached is equal to the rate at which they are regenerated (Figure 9.6).

*GMP is guanosine 5′-monophosphate, a unit of deoxyribonucleic acid (DNA).

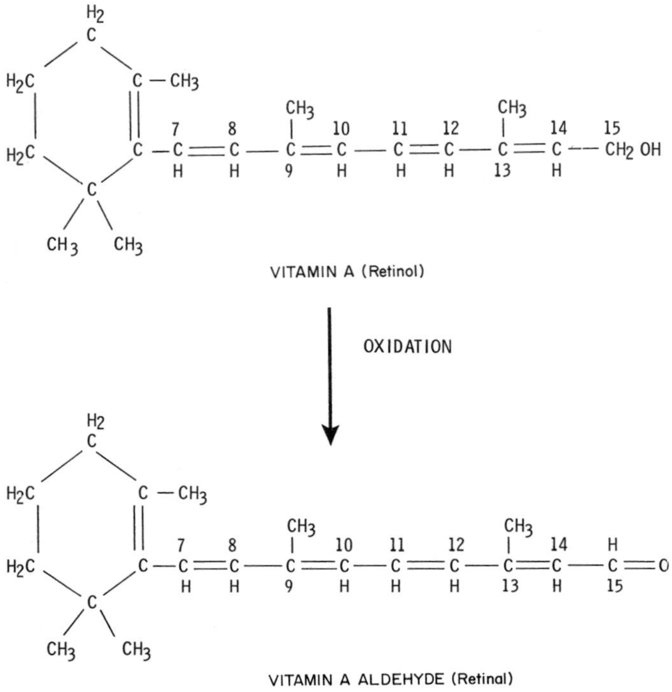

VITAMIN A (Retinol)

OXIDATION

VITAMIN A ALDEHYDE (Retinal)

Figure 9.4 Structural change of retinol upon oxidation to retinal.

FLOW CONDUCTIVITY AND RETINAL ADHESION

The attachment of the retina to the underlying tissue is not completely understood. We know that the loosest attachment is between the neural retina and the RPE because retinoschisis (splitting) and retinal detachment commonly occur between these layers rather than between the RPE and Bruch's membrane. Zauberman and Berman (1969) conducted a simple experiment to see if retinal adhesion was measurable. Strips of cat eye extending from the ora serrata to the optic disk were isolated and the force needed to peel the retina off the underlying tissue was recorded. When these strips were 5 mm wide, the force required to detach the retina at a rate of 5 mm/min was 50 to 90 mg over the tapetum lucidum and 120 to 250 mg over the tapetum nigrum. The required force was later found to increase directly with the peeling rate in rabbit eyes (deGuillebon and Zauberman 1972).

Kita and co-workers (1990) found the adhesive force of a normal rabbit retina was about 1.8×10^2 dynes/cm. Earlier, Marmor and associates (1980) had found that the peeling force was equivalent to 49 dyne/cm, and deGuillebon and Zauberman (1972) had found a value of about 60 to 150 dyne/cm (both also in rabbit eyes).

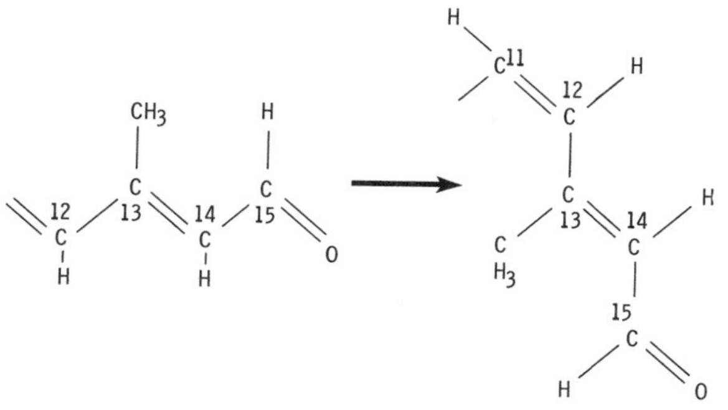

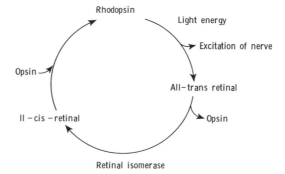

Figure 9.5 Isomerization of all-*trans*-retinal to all-*cis*-retinal.

Figure 9.6 Cycle showing rhodopsin bleaching and its regeneration. "Excitation" refers to excitation of the photoreceptors.

The semisolid vitreous cannot be the principal support because its liquefaction in middle age does not directly lead to retinal detachment. It is believed, however, that traction from condensing vitreous strands can overcome retinal attachment locally, leading to breaks and tears.

There is evidence that fluid pressure provides some support to the retina because *rhegmatogenous* retinal detachment occurs after a break or tear appears in the retina. Furthermore, when a tear in the retina is sealed, reattachment can occur without further intervention. Maurice, Salmon, and Zauberman (1971) indicated that IOP is usually low in eyes with detached retinas—and only after the break is sealed and the retina completely reattached does IOP return to a normal level. They attempted to measure the pressure difference across the retina, to support the postulate that internal pressure keeps the retina in its place, but no pressure difference (if present) was detected.

It appears that retinal adhesion is complex, related to a combination of metabolic and physical factors. It can be altered by a variety of conditions including temperature, pH, extracellular ions, and chemicals such as ouabain, cyanide, and acetazolamide (Endo et al. 1988; Yao et al. 1989). Although no direct physical connection has been found (Michaels et al 1990), it has been suggested that a viscous GAG-protein material "glues" the RPE to the photoreceptors. Some additional metabolic system enhances attachment, however, because adhesion is known to be reduced within minutes of enucleation or death. This metabolic system is believed to be related to the ability of the RPE cells to remove water from the subretinal space, transferring this fluid actively into the choroid (Miller et al. 1982). An example of such a pump mechanism is shown in Figure 9.7; ions are removed from the subretinal space by active transport, and the transfer of water follows osmotically to the choroid. Rates of RPE fluid transfer have been measured at 12 to 36 μl/cm^2 hour in mammals (Frambach and Marmor 1982; Negi and Marmor 1986; Cantrill and Pederson 1984) and 4 to 6 μl/cm^2 hour in frogs (Hughes et al. 1984).

Another force that may contribute to the attachment between the retina and underlying tissues has been termed *hydraulic drag*. This explanation for retinal adhesion uses the tube-type tire as a model. The neural retina is the inner tube and is pressed against its "casing," the underlying pigment epithelium, choroid, and sclera, by the internal pressure. The model requires that the retina be perfectly impermeable to the internal fluid; one can easily visualize that an inner tube made of sieve-like cheesecloth would not be pressed against the inner side of a tire casing whether the casing was air-tight or slightly permeable.

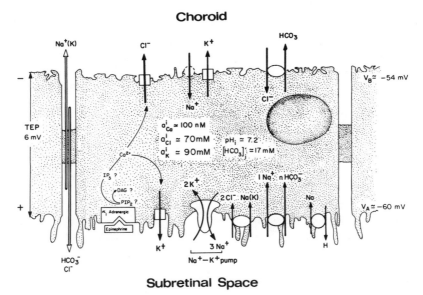

Figure 9.7 Schematic diagram of bovine retinal pigment epithelium and pathways for passive ionic flow and active transport of ions. Accompanying fluid transport (water) from the subretinal space through the pigment epithelial cell and into the choroid is also shown. (Courtesy of Sheldon S. Miller, PhD, University of California, Berkeley.)

Soft biological tissues, however, are never completely impermeable to water. But does the combination of fluids and tissues that make up the eye have properties that would lead to retinal adhesion even though this inner-tube model is not a complete and wholly satisfactory one?

Fatt and Shantinath (1971) measured both retinal density and flow conductivity (rabbit eyes) and found that tissue properties were consistent with the tube model of retinal adhesion. Data were collected on both fresh eyes (enucleated within 5 minutes of death and used immediately) and eyes that had been stored in the deep freeze ($-17°C$) for several weeks. (There was no noticeable difference in results between these groups, so these authors also concluded that storage at $-17°C$ did not affect these two tissue values.)

Density Measurement

Density measurements were made by the buoyancy method using two different solutions. First, a piece of fresh retina, about 5 mm square, was dropped into distilled water. A saturated solution of sucrose was immediately added (dropwise) until neutral buoyancy was obtained. A sample of this solution was then transferred to a refractometer. The observed refractive index was converted to specific gravity by use of tables of solution properties. With this method, it was noted that the retinal sample would sink after several minutes of neutral buoyancy. Neutral buoyancy could be reestablished by adding more sucrose to make the surrounding solution more dense. This behavior could be a result of osmotic withdrawal of water from the tissue by the sucrose solution. However, the dehydration process appeared to be slow, requiring several minutes to have an effect on tissue density. The neutral buoyancy obtained after less than 1 minute in the the solution probably represented the tissue in its original condition or very close to it.

To check this conclusion, density measurements were repeated on previously frozen retinal samples, using a hydrocarbon flotation liquid: namely, a mixture of iso-octane (density 0.70 gm/cm^3) and carbon tetrachloride (density 1.60 gm/cm^3). After separation under saline from the choroid, a retinal sample was touched to absorbent tissue paper to draw off any excess water. The sample was then dropped into the iso-octane, and carbon tetrachloride was added dropwise until neutral buoyancy was obtained. Under these conditions, samples were observed to remain at neutral buoyancy for at least 30 minutes. The specific gravity of this neutral buoyancy solution was obtained by weighing in a precalibrated 25-cm^3 pychometer bottle. The density of fresh and frozen rabbit retina was found to be 1.0174 ± 0.0007 gm/cm^3 by both methods.

Flow Conductivity Measurement

Flow conductivity was measured by passing isotonic saline through a 5-mm square piece of retina held on a fine screen as shown in Figure 9.8. The observed conductivity was that of the retina and the fine screen in series. The conductivity of the screen alone was determined in a separate set of flow conductivity experiments in which there was no retina attached, and then Equation 6.17 was used to determine the k/μ of the retina. For these calculations, the area of the open screen could be measured directly, and the thickness of the sample was assumed to be the value given by Prince (1964), namely 120 μm.

Table 9.1 shows the observed flow conductivity of rabbit retina and compares this value with those of other ocular tissues from the literature, stated in the usual flow conductivity units.

The density and flow conductivity data can be used to construct a modified inner-tube model of retinal adhesion. Let us assume that an eye is gazing downward at a 45° angle to the vertical plane, as shown in Figure 9.9. It is well known that a torn flap of the retina will usually return to the supporting tissue if the patient is lying horizontal, face upward. This must mean that the retina, with a density of 1.0174 gm/cm³, is more dense than the vitreous. The density of the vitreous can be approximated by assuming that this material is 99% water and 1% collagen (Pirie 1969); if the density of collagen is 1.33 gm/cm³, and the density of water is known (1.0 gm/cm³), the vitreous density (assuming volume additivity) may be calculated to be about 1.0033 gm/cm³.

The downward force, assuming that the retina is 0.1 mm thick and has no structural attachment to the underlying tissue, is 0.000141 gm/cm² of retina. How fast will this section of retina fall into a liquefied vitreous if all the liquid must pass through the section of retina that is falling? This problem is analogous to a porous

Table 9.1 Flow Conductivity of Rabbit Eye Tissues

	Retina*		
	Fresh	*Frozen*	*Mean*
Flow conductivity (cm⁴ dyn⁻¹ sec⁻¹ at 37°)	7.4×10^{-9}, 11.5×10^{-9}	7.4×10^{-9}, 8.4×10^{-9}, 12.3×10^{-9}, 24.6×10^{-9}, 45.6×10^{-9}	9.4×10^{-9} S.D. = 2.3×10^{-9}

	Sclera†	*Stroma‡*	*Epithelium§*	*Endothelium§*	*Descemet's membrane¶*	*Lens capsule #*
Flow conductivity (cm⁴ dyn⁻¹ sec⁻¹ at 37°)	19×10^{-13} (hydration = 2.14 gm H₂O per gm dry)	17.3×10^{-13} (hydration = 3.5 gm H₂O per gm dry)	0.27×10^{-13}	0.078×10^{-13}	1.95×10^{-13}	steer, 09.8×10^{-13}; calf, 1.12×10^{-13}

*The two largest values were not used in calculating the average because it was believed that a hole or thin sample could lead to high values. The two largest values are 6.6 and 16 times a standard deviation from the mean of the other five values.
†Fatt and Hedbys 1970b.
‡Hedbys and Mishima 1961.
§Mishima and Hedbys 1967.
¶Fatt 1969a.
#Fels 1970.
From Fatt and Shantinath (1971).

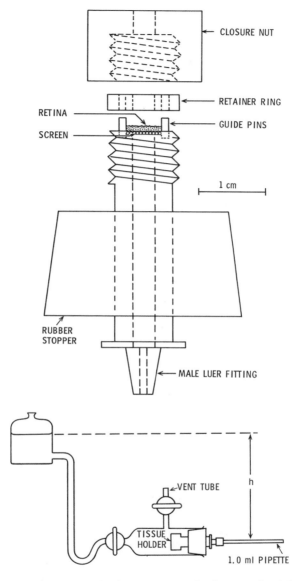

Figure 9.8 *Top*, cell and tissue holder for measuring the flow conductivity of the retina. All parts except guide pins, screen, and Luer fitting are of plastic. *Bottom*, flow apparatus for retina measurements. All parts except tissue holder and tube from supply bottle are made of glass. (With permission from Fatt I, Shantinath K [1971]: Flow conductivity of retina and its role in retinal adhesion. Exp. Eye Res. 12:218. Copyright by Academic Press Inc. [London] Ltd.)

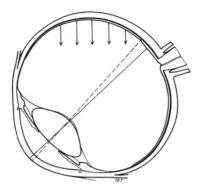

Figure 9.9 Eyeball in 45° downward gaze showing a section of retina that has a downward force because retina density is greater than density of the liquefied vitreous body. (With permission from Fatt I, Shantinath K [1971]: Flow conductivity of retina and its role in retinal adhesion. Exp. Eye Res. 12:218. Copyright by Academic Press Inc. [London] Ltd.)

piston problem, demonstrated in Figure 9.10. The problem is solved by taking the downward force as the weight of a square centimeter of retina after correction for buoyancy and then using Darcy's law to calculate how fast a water-like vitreous humor would pass through this tissue section. If the mean k/μ from Table 9.1 is used, it would take about 10 days for a 1-cm^2 section of the retina positioned as in Figure 9.10 to move down 1 mm, that is, to allow 0.1 cm^3 of water to pass through this section. It is clear that, unless the eye is held in a fixed position for very long periods of time, the intact retina cannot move away from the underlying tissue because of the long time it takes for the vitreous humor to move through the retina. Since gravity is the driving force in the calculation made above, it is also clear that sections of the retina below a horizontal meridian of an eye in horizontal gaze have no detaching force at all. A break in the superior retina invalidates these calculations by allowing the vitreous humor to pass through it directly, and there is then little or no resistance to movement of the retina away from the underlying tissue.

The only force acting on the retina in the above calculations is gravity. However, there may be another force, one that is uniform in all directions and pressing all portions of the retina toward the underlying tissues. Although the geometry of the eye is complex, an approximate calculation can be made by assuming that the vitreous has liquefied or, alternatively, that there is a film of liquid at the vitreous–retina interface that is hydraulically connected to the aqueous humor and is at intraocular pressure. By placing the retina and sclera in series, and from their known flow conductivities, the decrease in IOP across each tissue can be calculated. Fatt and Hedbys (1970b) determined the flow conductivity of the normal sclera (rabbit or human): 19×10^{-13} cm^4/dyne sec (37°C). The mean flow conductivity of retina is 9.4×10^{-9} (see Table 9.1). The thickness of

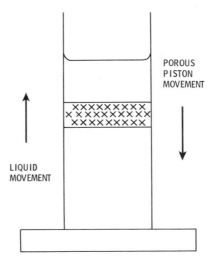

Figure 9.10 Model of a section of retina acting as a porous piston in a vertical cylinder. (With permission from Fatt I, Shantinath K [1971]: Flow conductivity of retina and its role in retinal adhesion. Exp. Eye Res. 12:210. Copyright by Academic Press Inc. [London] Ltd.)

human sclera can be taken as 0.06 cm, and that of the retina is estimated, as above, as 0.01 cm. The resistance to flow per unit area in the sclera is therefore (6 $\times$ 10^{-2})/(19 $\times$ 10^{-13}) dynes sec/cm^2, whereas across the retina the resistance to flow per unit area is (10^{-2})/(9.4 $\times$ 10^{-9}) dynes sec/cm^2. The total IOP of 18 mmHg will proportion itself across the layers such that 0.6 $\times$ 10^{-3} mmHg will be the pressure drop across the retina, the remainder being across the sclera. This is equivalent to a force of 0.00071 gm/cm^2. At first sight, this force appears very small, but it must be noted that the downward force of a section of retina was calculated above to be only 0.000141 gm/cm^2. It is apparent, therefore, that the hydraulic drag on the retina as aqueous or vitreous humor flows out of the eye via the uveoscleral route is 5 times greater than the gravitational force pulling the retina from the upper portions of the globe. Such a small pressure drop across the retina explains why Maurice, Salmon, and Zauberman (1971) were unable to detect any difference in pressure between the anterior chamber and a needle positioned under the retina.

The explanation for retinal adhesion given above leads to the conclusion that retinal detachment is likely only when a break is formed or when liquid leaks from the choroidal tissue behind the retina. Simple reduction of IOP is unlikely to reduce substantially the forces pressing the retina against the underlying tissues. A retinal break, however, allows fluid from the vitreous chamber to move freely behind the neural retina, thereby removing the pressure drop across this tissue.

This is in disagreement, however, with the results of Zauberman and de Guillebon (1972), who could not find experimental support for this theory of retinal adhesion. They found that retinal adhesion, as measured by the force needed to pull the retina off the pigment epithelium, was not affected by nearby breaks in the retina. They also found that retinal adhesion was much greater in the eye of a living animal than in its contralateral eye after death; thus they concluded that adhesion is dependent on the vitality of the cellular layers and did not attribute any role to IOP.

10

The Tears and the Lids

The tears and lids serve the eye in many different but important ways. Although there have been studies of tear flow, tear chemistry, tear film stability, and lid activity, much is still unknown. The variation in blinking rate among mammals, for example, is difficult to explain. Humans blink every 5 seconds, whereas the rabbit, with very much the same ocular physiological processes, blinks only once in 10 minutes. It is difficult to devise an explanation for the relation of blinking to tear film stability that permits such wide range in blinking rate.

THE TEARS
Function

The tear layer serves several purposes. The most important function of the tear film is to form an almost perfectly smooth optical surface on the cornea. Its second purpose is to serve as a lubricant for the eye and lids as the lids move over the exposed surface of the eye. A third function is to provide bactericidal action as a protection of the sensitive corneal epithelium. The enzyme lysozyme in the tears can destroy bacteria that enter the tear film. This bacteriolytic action is considered by some to be an important barrier to eye infection.

The tear film, of course, serves to keep the surface of the cornea moist. It is unlikely that the sensitive epithelial cells could survive if the surface were dry. The anteriorly directed movement of water through the cornea from the aqueous humor is not rapid enough to maintain a moist epithelial surface (see Chapter 6).

Film Structure

The tear film on the eye has been subdivided into three separate layers: the outermost oily layer, the central aqueous phase, and a layer of mucin (large molecules that are glycoproteins with a large amount of carbohydrate) in contact with the epithelial surface (Holly 1973). The thickness of the oily layer varies with the width of the palpebral fissure. The film is normally between 50 and 500 nm thick. Oil films of this thickness are at least two molecules thick.

Figure 10.1 shows the oily layer as a heavy dark line on the underlying aqueous layer. As the lids close, moving from right to left in the figure, the oily layer thickens until it is shown as wrinkled. The reader can verify this effect by closing the lids to the minimum slit width that allows light from a bright source to enter the eye. The entopic view of the tear film shows moving strands that are parallel to the edge of the upper and lower lids. As the lids are separated the strands clear from the central field of vision but are still seen near the lids.

The aqueous phase of the tear film is a dilute water solution of salts and dissolved organic materials. The water content is 98.2%, with 1.8% dissolved solids. The concentration of the various inorganic dissolved solids is given in Table 10.1 together with the concentrations in other fluids for comparison. The dissolved organic material in the aqueous phase is composed of glycoproteins (Berta and Török 1986). The aqueous layer is from 6 to 7 μm thick, but the thickness may be greater during excessive lacrimation (crying) (Mishima and Maurice 1961a, b).

At the interface between the aqueous layer and the epithelium is a viscous, sticky material called the *mucoid layer,* which is about 20 to 40 nm thick. The mucoid material is a combination of glycoproteins and glycosaminoglycans (GAGs) produced by conjunctival goblet cells. In the rabbit there appear to be three separate GAGs with molecular weights of 14,000, 50,000, and 400,000. The mucoid layer is believed to help spread the aqueous phase of the tears over the lipid-like surface of the epithelial cells. The structure of the GAG molecule enables

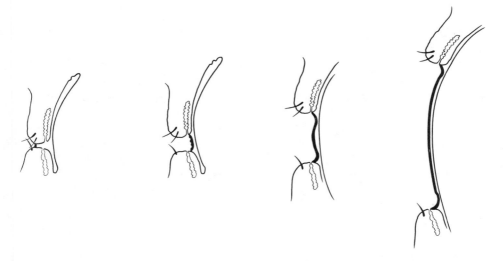

Figure 10.1   The tear layer between the lids is covered with an oily layer, shown as a dark band. At right the eye is fully open. As the eye is closed, from right to left, the oily layer becomes compressed until it becomes wrinkled when the lids are separated by only a millimeter.

Table 10.1 Concentration of Inorganic Ions in Ocular Fluids*

Species	Fluid	Concentration (µEq/ml)			
		Na +	*K +*	*Cl⁻*	*HCO₃⁻*
Rabbit	Tears	149	17	131	20
		151	29	138	—
		137.5	15.3	136.6	—
		147.1	13.8	132.8	—
	Serum	146	4	111	22
		—	—	106.2*	25.7*
		151.1*	5.50*	—	27.4*
	Aqueous humor	153.1	—	105.7	30.9
		138	5.0	101.0	30.2
		143.5	5.25	—	33.6
Human	Tears	146	16.2	128	—
		145	24.1	128	26
		144.4	19.3	144.9	—
	Serum	136–145	4.1–5.6	98–106	21–30
		139–148	3.6–5.0	98–106	25–32*
		—	—	107.0*	27.5*
	Aqueous humor	—	—	131.0	20.15*

*In plasma.

*From Iwata S (1973): Chemical composition of the aqueous phase. In Holly FJ, Klemp MA (eds): The Preocular Tear Film and Dry Eye Syndromes. International Ophthalmology Clinics. Boston, Little, Brown.

it to attach itself to the epithelial cell surface and at the same time be soluble in the aqueous layer of the tear film. Particles from the air and cellular debris from the epithelium collect at the mucin–aqueous interface and are then swept by lid action into the inferior fornix (Norn 1969; Fatt 1991).

Sources of the Tear Film Components

The aqueous phase of the tear film is produced in the lacrimal glands and in the accessory glands of Krause and Wolfring (Figures 10.2 and 10.3). These glands produce a liquid that is truly a secretion and not merely a filtrate of the blood plasma.

The oily material that covers the surface of the tear film is produced by the meibomian glands and the gland of Moll (see Figure 10.3), both in the upper lid.

The mucoid material that forms the interface between the aqueous tear layer and the epithelium is produced in the conjunctival goblet cells found throughout the conjunctiva, particularly in the fornices. These cells occur in the conjunctival epithelium, where they grow to a large size as mucoid material accumulates inside the cell. The cell then migrates to the surface, where it ruptures and discharges the mucoid material into the tears. The remaining parts of the cell then degenerate.

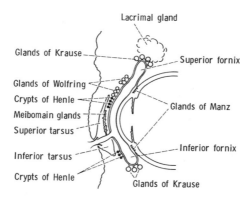

Figure 10.2 Diagrammatic representation of a sagittal section through the eyelids and eyeball showing the conjuctival sac and the position of its glands.

This process of forming and discharging a glandular secretion is called *holocrine* secretion.

Composition of the Tear Film

The aqueous part of the tear film forms by far the largest part of the tear liquid. The continuous evaporation of water from the tears makes defining a "tear composition" very difficult. A second confusing factor is the sensitivity of the tear-producing processes to stimulation while the tears are being collected for analysis.

Iwata (1973) compares the concentration of inorganic ions in the tears with concentrations in other body fluids in Table 10.1. These concentrations are presumably for freshly produced tears. Evaporation between blinks may raise all of the concentrations by 10% to 20%. Also, Iwata's data must be assumed to be for tears produced without external stimulation.

In addition to the GAGs (already mentioned as present in the aqueous phase), there are small amounts of low-molecular-weight organic materials in the tears. Glucose is present in a concentration of about 3 to 10 mg/ml. This concentration is one-tenth of the concentration in the blood serum. There is no evidence that corneal cells can use glucose when present at the very low concentration found in the tears. The concentration of urea in the tears is about the same as in the blood plasma, about 54 mg per 100 ml. A small amount of amino acids, 8 mg per 100 ml, is also present. High-molecular-weight proteinaceous materials appear in the tears at a concentration of between 0.3% and 0.7% in humans. In rabbit tears the concentration may be as high as 1.3%. The protein types are shown in Table 10.2. The function of albumin and globulin in the tears is not known. Andrews (1970) believes that the albumin aids the oily meibomian secretion in stabilizing the thin tear film. The lysozyme acts as a bactericidal agent for protection of the epithelium.

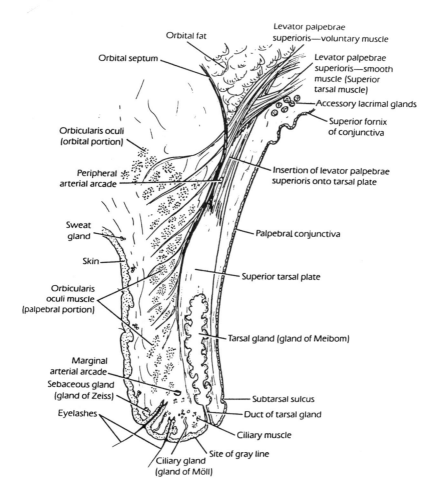

Figure 10.3 Detailed anatomy of the upper lid. (From Snell RS, Lemp MS [1989]: Clinical Anatomy of the Eye. Boston, Blackwell. With permission.)

Table 10.2 Types of Protein*

Fractions	Unstimulated (Normal) Flow (%)	Stimulated Flow (%)
Albumin	58.2	20.2
Globulin	23.9	56.9
Lysozyme	17.9	22.9

*From Iwata S (1973): Chemical composition of the acqueous phase. In Holly FJ, Klemp MA (eds): The Preocular Tear Film and Dry Eye Syndromes. International Ophthalmology Clinics. Boston, Little, Brown.

The lipogenous meibomian secretion is a low melting point mixture of cholesterol ester and lecithin with minor amounts of fatty acids. The meibomian secretion collected directly from the gland is a solid or semisolid at room temperature. It has a melting point that is in the range 35° to 40°C (Brown and Dervichian 1969). At 40°C the secretion is a liquid. The bulk of the secretion is a nonpolar hydrocarbon that by itself would not spread over the aqueous tear layer. A surface-active component, a molecule with a hydrophilic end chain, present in the secretion spreads on the aqueous layer and carries with it the bulk of the lipid component.

Holly (1973) combines all of the tear components into a tear film that has four distinct layers. He distributes some of the mucoid material (mucin) through the tear film to give the picture shown in Figure 10.4. The mucin coacervate layer has mucin molecules that have formed submicroscopic-size liquid aggregates. The existence of a four-layer aqueous film, as pictured by Holly in Figure 10.4, is not consistent with the hypothesis of circulation in the tear prism of the lid margin during blinking. Further description of tear circulation in the margin is given below when lid motion is treated.

Stability of the Tear Film

The tears can function properly only if the tear film covers the entire eye and is reestablished quickly and completely after a blink. In the normal human eye the tear film is complete, that is, without holes, during the 5-second period between blinks. If, however, the eye is held open, either voluntarily or by force, the tear film ruptures after 15 to 40 seconds and dry spots appear on the cornea. It is of interest to note that among the lower animals the tear film can remain complete for as long as 600 seconds between blinks.

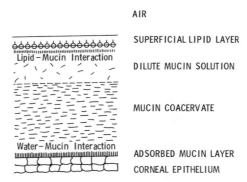

Figure 10.4 A proposed structure of the tear film. (From Holly FJ [1973]: Formation and stability of the tear film. In Holly FJ, Lemp MA [eds]: The Preocular Tear Film and Dry Eye Syndromes, Vol. 13, No. 1. International Ophthalmology Clinics. Boston, Little, Brown.)

Rupture of the tear film after 15 to 40 seconds cannot be the result of evaporation because at least 10 minutes is required to evaporate away the aqueous phase of the tear film while the oily layer is in place. Holly (1973) pictures the break in the tear film taking place as shown in Figure 10.5. In the Holly picture the tear film thins uniformly by evaporation. When the tear film has thinned to some critical thickness, a significant number of lipid molecules begin to be attracted by the mucoid layer and migrate down to this layer. The migration process is enhanced if there is any spontaneous local thinning. When the mucoid layer on the epithelium is sufficiently contaminated by lipid migrating down from the top surface of the tear layer, the mucoid becomes hydrophobic and the tear film ruptures. Blinking can supposedly repair the rupture by removing the lipid contaminant from the mucoid layer and restoring a thick aqueous layer.

This mechanism for tear film break-up, usually known as the Holly or Holly and Lemp mechanism, has had widespread acceptance even though there is little direct evidence of its validity. Furthermore, close examination of the mechanism shows that there are several features that contradict what is known about thin water films. The thinning of the aqueous layer required to allow molecular attraction of the lipid molecules to the mucin layer on the epithelium would reduce the tensile strength of the aqueous layer to the point where suction forces from the tear fluid meniscii at the upper and lower lid margins would break the thin water

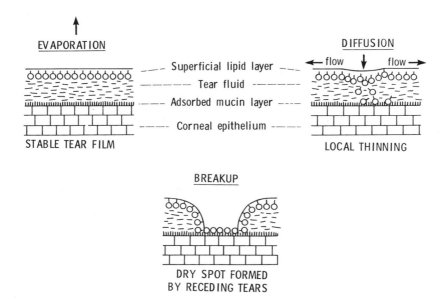

Figure 10.5 Hypothetical mechanism for tear film break-up. (From Holly FJ [1973]: Formation and stability of the tear film. In Holly FJ, Lemp MA [eds]: The Preocular Tear Film and Dry Eye Syndromes, Vol. 13, No. 1. International Ophthalmology Clinics. Boston, Little, Brown.)

film. There is then no need to hypothesize development of hydrophobicity of the mucin layer.

A second deficiency of the Holly and Lemp picture of tear film break-up is its inability to explain the consequence of continuous periodic break-up. Most persons suffering from abnormal tear film break-up are not disabled by formation of a lipid-coated epithelium. In the Holly and Lemp picture, closure of the lids over the lipid already deposited on the epithelium should deposit more lipid. The final outcome of many blinks would be a cornea totally covered by lipid and consequently a disabled eye. This outcome is not seen among patients suffering from abnormal tear film break-up.

An alternative to the Holly and Lemp picture of tear film break-up can be developed by starting with the McDonald and Brubaker (1971) description of meniscus-induced thinning of the tear film. Figure 10.6, from McDonald and Brubaker, shows bands of thinned tear film created by suction from the curved tear meniscii in the lid margins. These bands can be easily seen in an entopic view by observing a bright light through a pinhole. Light bands are from tears in the

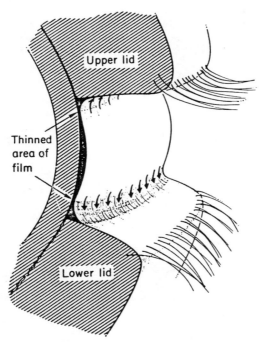

Figure 10.6 The McDonald-Brubaker model of tear film thinning. Negative pressure generated by the curved surface of the tear liquid prism in the lid margins thins the adjacent tear film. (From McDonald JE, Brubaker S [1971]: Meniscus-induced thinning of tear films. Am. J. Ophthalmol. 72:139–146. With permission from the American Journal of Ophthalmology. Copyright by the Ophthalmic Publishing Co.)

margins. The parallel dark lines are from thin bands of tear film that are about 1 mm away from the top and bottom lids. These bands normally disappear in a few seconds but can be observed for a minute or longer if a few drops of a viscosity-enhancing artificial tear fluid are added to the eye.

The existence of the thin bands of the McDonald-Brubaker picture indicates that there is drainage of tear liquid from the surface of the open eye. During the drainage period the tear fluid from the central area of the cornea must pass through the thin bands on its way to the lid margins. Since the bands are thin they offer a high resistance to liquid flow, thereby providing a mechanism that slows tear drainage from the cornea.

The lids can be held open manually until the tear film breaks. At the break point the suction from the tears in the lid margin has thinned the tears on the cornea to the point where the tensile strength of this thin water layer is less than the suction force created by the meniscii in the lid margins. This picture of tear film break-up does not use either lipid or mucin in the break-up mechanism. The absence of a lipid layer may allow faster evaporation, thereby allowing the aqueous tear film to arrive sooner at a thickness where suction forces from the margin will break the film but the lipid has played no direct role in the tear film break-up. In studies on plastic model eyes (Fatt, 1991) a coating of mucin on the plastic eye was found to lead to a thinner water layer at break-up. An interaction between the water-soluble groups on the mucin and the water layer is postulated as the mechanism for giving the water film greater tensile strength, but no detailed explanation for the phenomenon is available.

In the normal eye the tear film does not break between blinks. The blink, driven by some yet unknown reflex stimulus, takes place about 5 seconds after the lid has come to rest following the prior blink. The maximum downward velocity of the upper lid ranges from 12 cm/sec to 30 cm/sec (Hayashi 1977; Doane 1980). The maximum velocity is reached after the lid has traveled about 6 mm from its stationary upper position. Total travel of the upper lid is about 12 mm. A pictorial representation of the upper and lower lids in correct relative scale for the human eye is shown in Figure 10.7. In this sagittal section taken at the midpoint between the two canthii the lid is resting on the cornea along a line on the inside of the lid just below the subtarsal sulcus. The line of contact runs across the globe from canthus to canthus. Along this line the upper lid force of 2.5 to 5×10^3 dynes per cm^2 pressing against the globe reduces the tear film thickness to 0.5 to 1.0 μm (Hayashi 1977). As the lid moves downward over the globe it acts as a wiper, reducing the normal open-eye tear film thickness of 7 to 10 μm to 0.5 to 1.0 μm. The difference of tear film thickness of about 9 μm is pushed ahead of the lid. If the canthus-to-canthus distance is taken as 25 mm in the adult human eye, then for each 1-mm downward movement the upper lid sweeps ahead of itself 0.225 μl. After moving 3 mm, one-quarter of its total travel of 12 mm, the upper lid will have swept ahead of itself about 0.68 μl. At the half-way point, 1.32 μl will have been swept up, and at lid closure, 2.64 μl will collect in the narrow opening between the closed lids.

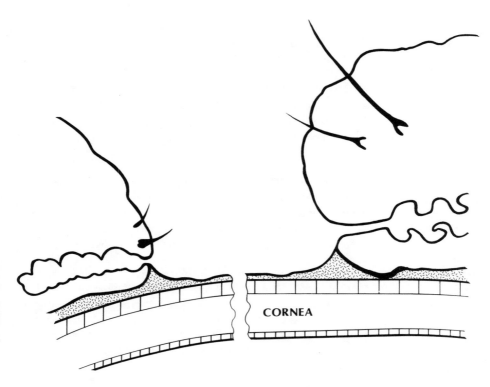

Figure 10.7 Tear film on the cornea of the open eye. Upper lid is on the right.

The question that must now be considered is where is the swept-up tear fluid stored until the lids open and spread the tears across the eye? There are several choices. The tear layer on the eye can uniformly increase in thickness. This would mean that when the lids are at the midpoint of closure, the tear film is about 15 to 20 μm thick uniformly over that part of the eye that is still open. Another possibility is that the lid pushes a narrow thick band of tears ahead of itself (Fatt 1991). Finally, the tears pushed ahead of the lid can be stored in the tear film prism in the lid margin.

The possibility of tear fluid storage in the tear prism of the lid margin can be subjected to further analysis through the use of data provided by Port and Asaria (1990). They reported an average prism height of 0.18 mm. Figure 10.7 shows that this height represents the height of an equilateral triangle with a base length that is about twice the height. The tear prism of the upper lid has a volume of 0.81 μl when the lid is fully retracted in the open-eye position. At the half-way point of closure we have seen that there are 1.32 μl to be stored. If all of this swept-up tear fluid is stored in the upper-lid tear prism then the prism height must be greater. The natural upper limit to the height of the prism is the gray line (intermarginal sulcus). At this line the skin of the lid changes from the highly water-wettable tissue of the palpebral conjunctiva to the less wettable skin of the anterior surface of the lid. The height of the gray line appears to be about 0.4 to 0.8 mm above the surface of the cornea. A prism of 0.4 to 0.8 mm high could store from 4 to 16 μl of tear fluid—far more than is swept up during lid closure. Although there is no experimental evidence, it is clear that the tear margin offers the space for storage of the tear fluid during lid closure.

Another fluid-movement feature of the tear prism is demonstrated in Figure 10.8. As the upper lid moves downward, from right to left in Figure 10.8, there is no relative motion of an infinitely thin tear layer on the cornea nor on the lid surface. This concept of no liquid motion of the layer in contact with a solid is standard in all fluid mechanics when treating liquid flow problem in the laminar flow range, that is, at low velocities. Lid motion is in the velocity range where laminar flow is expected. As shown in Figure 10.8 there is lid motion with respect to the cornea; therefore the layer of tear fluid adjacent to the lid is moving with respect to the cornea. Under these conditions there will be a circulation of tear fluid, as shown by the curved arrow in Figure 10.8. This circulation would be expected to make the tear fluid well mixed under the lipid layer. A well-mixed tear fluid could not maintain the layering of mucin into a layer of coacervate under a layer of dilute mucin solution as proposed by Holly and shown here in Figure 10.4.

In Figure 10.6 the eye has been open for about 5 seconds. The bands of thin tear film parallel to the lids have prevented the central portion of the tear film from thinning below the 10-μm thickness usually reported as tear film thickness.

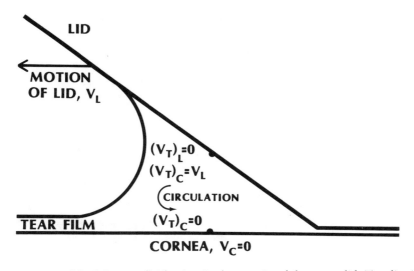

Figure 10.8 Model of the tear fluid prism in the margin of the upper lid. Tear liquid is attached to the lid and cornea, as indicated by dots on the lid and cornea. As the lid moves to the left, tear liquid in contact with the lid is dragged with it. The liquid in contact with the cornea remains stationary. Circulation in the tear prism is a consequence of the shearing forces applied to the tear liquid.

A rapidly downward moving upper lid may push tear film ahead of itself, but this wave will soon encounter the upper thin band (as shown in Figure 10.6). The thin band is obliterated by fluid pushed ahead by the lid. The lid continues moving downward across the globe until all of the liquid pushed ahead is collected between the lids, some as prisms in the upper and lower lid margins and some filling the space between the lids.

In Figure 10.1 a thick layer of tear fluid is shown between the lids in the almost closed eye. This layer has a wrinkled film of lipid at its surface. The surface is concave, as shown in Figure 10.1. The concave nature of the surface can easily be verified by closing the lids until only a slit remains open and then viewing a vertical thin object or interface between light and dark, such as the edge of a window frame when light is coming in through the window. Tilting the head causes the vertical line to bend, indicating that the line is being viewed through a cylindrical lens.

The maximum upward velocity of the upper lid is, according to Doane (1980), about one-half of the downward velocity. At this velocity (in the range of 5 to 15 cm/sec) of separation of the lids, the lid margins pull tear fluid away from the central pool faster than the bulk of the tear fluid can travel. As a consequence the thin bands form parallel to the lids, trapping a central pool of tear fluid. In time the central pool will thin further as tear fluid is pulled through the thin bands, but the succeeding blink takes place before the central pool thins below 10 μm. When some investigators report tear film thickness greater than 10 μm they may be observing a trapped central pool that is thinning slowly because of special circumstances in the eye under study. On the other hand, a very slowly opening pair of lids may not give the McDonald-Brubaker bands and the thick central pool because the upper lid can slowly draw the tear fluid with itself to spread a uniformly thin tear film on the eye.

Tear Production Rate

The rate of tear production in the normal, unstimulated eye is difficult to measure because the approach of a sampling device stimulates abnormal lacrimation. In the Schirmer test used by optometrists and ophthalmologists, the end of a strip of absorbent paper is touched to the eye. The length of wetted zone is a measure of tear quantity in the eye. This test is only a very crude measure of tear production rate and leads to no numerical data.

Estimates of tear production rate can be made from the chemical composition of freshly produced tears, the composition of the steady-state tear film on the eye, and the rate of evaporation of the aqueous component of the tear film. The best estimate of normal tear production rate is 1.2 μl/min, although some authorities claim the rate is below 1 μl/min (Doane and Gleason 1991). Since the tear volume in the eye at any time is about 7 μl (Doane and Gleason 1991) the turnover rate is about once every 5 to 7 minutes. Abnormal lacrimation brought about by irritation or emotion can increase the production rate several hundredfold. The drainage mechanism is then overwhelmed and excess tears run down the cheek. One drop of tear fluid running down the cheek of a person who is crying contains 50 μl, and many of these drops can be produced each minute.

It is of interest to note that abnormal tearing starts only after an infant is 4 months old. A newborn produces no excess tear fluid even when crying loudly. The absence of excess tearing in very young infants may be connected with the low enervation of the cornea. A newborn can tolerate large particles on the cornea without being uncomfortable.

Evaporation and Temperature

Evaporation from the tear film is estimated to be about 10% of the production rate. That makes the evaporation rate 0.12 μl/min. There is little effect of air motion over the eye on evaporation rate because most of the resistance to evaporation is the oily layer on the tear-film surface rather than the stagnant zone of water-saturated air. If the oily layer is removed, or if the meibomian glands do not produce their secretion, evaporation is very rapid even in still air, and the eye will become dry between blinks.

Although one would expect evaporation to be an important factor in establishing tear temperature, in fact evaporation carries off only about 13% of heat lost from the surface of the eye. About 46% of the heat is carried away by convection, that is, by heat transfer directly to the surrounding air, and 41% by radiation. Radiative heat transfer is by means of transfer of heat energy in the form of electromagnetic waves in the infrared wavelength region from the warm eye to colder surfaces in the surrounding environment.

The corneal surface temperature, representing the temperature in the tear film, is shown in Figure 10.9 as a function of air temperature and air velocity. It is clear that a windy (10 mph, or 14 km/hour), cold ($-15°C$) environment can lower the tear temperature to such low levels, about 5°C, that metabolism in the epithelial cells will cease (Freeman and Fatt 1973).

THE LIDS

Earlier in this chapter some aspects of lid motion were described in connection with the formation and stability of the tear film. However, lid movement is of interest in itself because of the protection offered by a blink and because lid motion influences the performance of a contact lens.

The lids are a movable cover for the exposed portions of the eye. An anatomical description of the lids is given in Figures 1.8, 10.2, and 10.3. The lids have several functions. They protect the sensitive eye tissue. Any action that is interpreted as a possible danger to the eye elicits an immediate reflex blink reaction that closes the lids. The lids close the eye during sleep, thereby reducing the level of external stimuli reaching the nervous system. Finally, as has already been described in some detail, the lids serve to spread the tears uniformly over the eye so that a high-quality optical surface is maintained on the cornea.

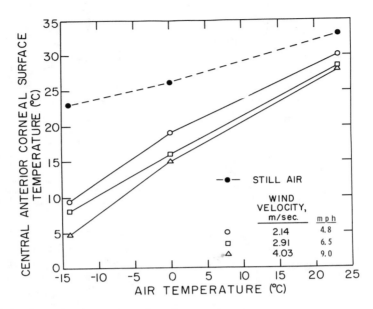

Figure 10.9 Central anterior corneal surface temperature, determined with a thermistor temperature sensor, as a function of ambient air temperature for various air velocities at the eye. (From Freeman RD, Fatt I [1973]: Environmental influences on ocular temperature. Invest. Ophthalmol. 12:596–602.)

Lid Activity

Although the need for an occasional blink is easy to explain in terms of tear renewal, it is much more difficult to explain the observed normal rate of involuntary periodic blinking. This blink rate varies from 12/min in humans to once every 10 or 15 minutes in the rabbit even though there is little or no difference in corneal physiology between these two species. Because the corneas are so much alike in humans and rabbits, some investigators have suggested that blinking is related to perception and that the relatively rapid blink rate in humans is part of the information-processing procedure of the retina and brain. As yet there is no good evidence for this hypothesis. The various kinds of lid activity are summarized in Table 10.3.

The involuntary reflex blink may be stimulated by strong light, loud noise, touching the cornea, or sudden and unexpected approach of an object toward the eye. In preparation for sleep, closure of the eyes may be voluntary or involuntary.

Detailed studies of lid motion have rarely been made. Gordon (1951) used a shutterless motion-picture camera to record the movement of a shiny steel ball glued to the upper lid. Brown and co-workers (1973) recorded the movement of the eyelid by the simple expedient of putting a photocell in place of the eyepiece in a biomicroscope. The difference in reflectivity between the eyelid and the cornea gave a varying electric signal from the photocell as the lid moved down

Table 10.3 Summary of Lid Activity

Type	Name	Function
Voluntary	Bilateral (blink)	Protective
	Unilateral (wink)	Communication; use of monocular instruments
Involuntary	Periodic blink	Replenishment of tear film
	Reflex blink	Protective

over the eye. A sample record from the study of Brown and associates is shown in Figure 10.10. The wavy signal superimposed on the blink is 60-Hz interference from power lines and serves as a time-base calibration. Figure 10.10 shows that this blink had an amplitude of about 9.5 mm. The amplitude varies from individual to individual and is affected by contact lens wear, as will be discussed later. In Doane's study (1980) of four individuals the maximum upper lid movement was 12 mm and the minimum was 5 mm. The length of the blink, from full open eye (upper part of trace in Figure 10.10) to full open after a blink is about 0.33 second. This is of course not the period of no vision because the lids do not cover the central optical zone of the pupil for this 0.33-second period.

Hayashi (1977) and Doane (1980) have used high-speed motion-picture photography to capture the details of lid motion. A frame-by-frame analysis yields the position of the lid as a function of time. Lid velocity can be derived from graphs of lid position as a function of time. Velocity can then be related to lid position and to time after the lid starts its descent.

Hayashi's results are summarized in Figure 10.11. Several interesting features of blinking are apparent in Figure 10.11. First, the downward movement of the upper lid is transmitted to the lower lid, and after contact the lower lid moves down. Second, the upper lid covers the center of the pupil for a period of 0.10 second. The time of total lost vision is probably not greater than 0.15 second. The loss of vision for 0.15 second may be serious for occupations that require close observation of rapid motion. For example, an airplane pilot whose airplane is moving at 600 mph (960 km/hour) or 880 feet/sec (300 m/sec) moves 132 feet (40 m) during the time he has no vision because the lids are blocking his pupils. He, of course, retains the image of his surroundings just before the lid blocked the pupils, but during 0.15 second he gains no new information. Third, there is a Bell's phenomenon; the pupil begins to move upward just before the upper lid reaches the center of the pupil.

Hayashi's study was carried out to observe contact lens movement in the eye during blinking. Figure 10.11 is therefore a good introduction to the effects of contact lenses on blinking. A similar study was made by Brown and co-workers (1973) who made less detailed measurement of lid movement but, instead, observed blinking period, amplitude, and duration for an eye wearing a hard contact lens (PMMA) or a soft, hydrogel lens. Their data are summarized in Table 10.4.

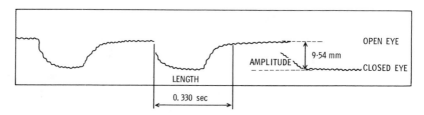

Figure 10.10 Sample recording of a blink. The maximum spacing between the lids was 9.54 mm, and the time from full open lid to return to full open is 0.330 seconds. (From Brown M, Chinn S, Fatt I, Harris MG [1973]: The effect of soft and hard contact lenses on blink rate, amplitude, and length. J. Am. Optom. Assoc. 44:254–257. Reprinted with permission of the Journal of the American Optometric Association.)

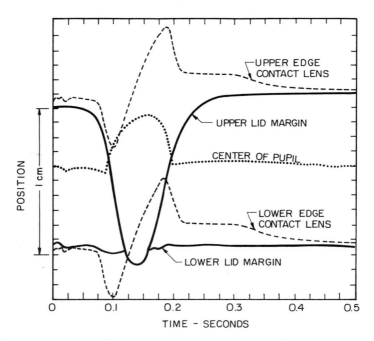

Figure 10.11 Movement of lids, center of pupil, and a hard contact lens on the cornea during a blink. (From Hayashi TT [1977]: Mechanics of contact lens motion. Ph.D. Thesis. Berkeley, University of California.)

Table 10.4 shows that of the three blink characteristics (amplitude, duration, and rate) the amplitude and the rate are significantly affected by a hard contact lens. Although this study was done with the older PMMA lenses there is no reason to believe that the results would have been any different with modern RGP hard lenses. The soft lens has no effect at all. Hayashi's more detailed study of lid and contact lens movement (Figure 10.11) shows that the contact lens is driven down

Table 10.4   Blink Characteristics

Blink Characteristics	Before Lens Insertion	After Soft Lens Insertion	After Hard Lens Insertion
Amplitude	4.84 mm ±0.80* (n = 13) 0.182 sec	3.04 mm ± 0.90 (n = 8) 0.216 sec	9.45 mm ± 1.45 (n = 4) 0.236 sec
Length	± 0.03 (n = 14) 15.8/min	±0.028 (n = 9) 17.5/min	±0.038 (n = 6) 9.75/min
Rate	± 7.9 (n = 13)	± 6.9 (n = 8)	± 5.4 (n = 5)

*Standard deviation. Differences between averages are not considered to be significant if they are less than two standard deviations of the average (defined as, $S_{av}^3 = \frac{2}{1} + \frac{2}{2}$).

*From Brown M, Chinn S, Fatt I, Harris MG (1973): The effect of soft and hard contact lenses on blink rate, amplitude, and length. J. Am. Optom. Assoc. 42:254–257.

by the downward movement of the upper lid until the bottom edge of the lens is about 3 mm below the lid margin. Then the upward movement of the eye carries the lens with it until the bottom edge of the lens is approximately at the center of the eye. The upper edge of the lens has meanwhile moved far under the upper lid. After the lid retracts, the lens is brought down with the eye and slowly floats down to its initial open-eye position.

The studies of Brown and co-workers (1973) and Hayashi (1977) are of interest because they show lid motion related to contact lens wear but there were so few subjects in their studies that the effect of intersubject variability could not be determined. Doane (1980) used refined methods of high-speed motion-picture photography to show details of lid motion for four subjects. Figure 10.12 from Doane (1980) shows that the repetitive blink characteristics for a given subject are very much the same, but there is great variation from one subject to another. In subject C maximum lid velocity was about 30 cm/sec, whereas in subject D it was 12 cm/sec. Also, in subjects A and C each blink has about the same characteristic pattern, but in subjects B and D each blink is different. In B, for example, some blinks have a maximum velocity of almost 30 cm/sec but only 17 cm/sec for others.

It must be pointed out that all lid velocities are for the point on the lid midway between the canthii. At this point lid velocity is a maximum, measured as a linear velocity on the surface of the globe. This velocity decreases from the midpoint to each canthus where the lid velocity is zero.

The upper lid reaches its maximum velocity just as it crosses the optic axis of the eye, and then the lid decelerates. Doane found that the upper lid sometimes came to rest before touching the lower lid. The upward movement of the lid is always slower than the downward movement. The maximum upward velocity is usually one-half of the maximum downward velocity.

Doane (1980) has devised a table, reproduced here as Table 10.5, in which he has averaged results from 10 subjects to arrive at what he calls a "standard blink."

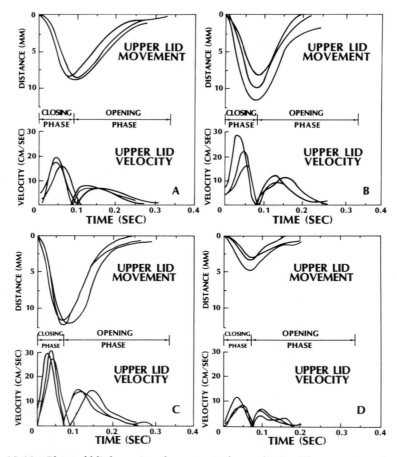

Figure 10.12 Plots of blink motion dynamics in four subjects. The upper set of curves of each pair represents the time course of the upper lid displacement during the closing and opening phases. The lower set of curves is the time course of the instantaneous velocity of the upper lid, which is zero at the point where the lid reverses direction. Note variation between individuals. Subject *D, lower right graph,* had a narrow palpebral fissure, and consequently the lid excursions and velocities are less than normal. (From Doane MG [1980]: Interaction of eyelids and tears in corneal wetting and the dynamics of the normal human eye blink. Am. J. Ophthalmol. 89:507–516. With permission from the American Journal of Ophthalmology. Copyright by the Ophthalmic Publishing Co.)

Table 10.5 Dynamics of Upper Eyelid Motion During a Blink*

Factor	Value†	
Duration of closing phase	82.1	±2.1 msec
Duration of opening phase	175.8	±11.0 msec
Total blink duration	257.9	11.3 msec
Maximum closing velocity	18.7	1.7 cm/sec
Maximum opening velocity	9.7	0.7 cm/sec

*From Doane MG (1980): Interaction of eyelids and tears in corneal wetting and the dynamics of the normal human eyeblink. Am. J. Ophthalmol. 89:507–516. With permission from the American Journal of Ophthalmology. Copyright by the Ophthalmic Publishing Co.

†Each value given is an average of 40 blinks ± standard error of the mean in 10 different subjects.

The lower lid has only horizontal motion. This motion is directed toward the medial canthus as the upper lid moves downward and then temporally as the lid moves upward. Both Hayashi and Doane have seen a slight, 1-mm downward movement of the lower lid as the upper lid touches it. The horizontal movement of the lower lid serves to move tear fluid and any debris it may have entrained toward the medial canthus, where it can be drained from the eye via the punctal openings.

The upward rotation of the globe during a blink is known as *Bell's phenomenon*. There is some controversy over the conditions needed to elicit Bell's phenomenon. Hayashi's graphical display of lid, pupil, and contact lens movement, given here in Figure 10.11, shows a 5-mm upward displacement of the center of the pupil during a blink. Doane and Gleason (1991), however, claim that only a forced blink elicits Bell's phenomenon. They quote Duke-Elder and Scott (1971), who said ". . . in voluntary closure the upward rotation varies in extent directly with the amount of energy expended in the act of closure, being absent when little effort is required." Doane and Gleason remark that little effort is expended during normal, unconscious blinking and therefore there should be little or no Bell's phenomenon. On the other hand, a simple observation made of the moving spot on a cathode ray oscilloscope screen shows that there is some upward eye rotation during the minimally forced voluntary blink. If the sweep rate of the oscilloscope is running at 100 cm/sec, a downward displacement of the trace is seen during a voluntary blink. This shift of the trace must indicate an upward rotation of the globe.

Doane (1980) has also observed an inward movement of the globe during a blink. The globe moves inward in step with the descent of the upper lid. When the lids are fully closed the globe has moved inward about 1.5 mm.

References

Adler VA, Cringle SJ, Constable IJ (1983): The retinal oxygen profile in cats. Invest. Ophthalmol. Vis. Sci. 24:30–36.

Allansmith M, de Ramus A, Maurice DM (1979): The dynamics of IgG in the cornea. Invest. Ophthalmol. Vis. Sci. 18:947–955.

Andrews JS (1970): Human tear film lipids. I. Composition of the principal nonpolar components. Exp. Eye Res. 10:223–227.

Ang JHB, Efron N (1989): Carbon dioxide permeability of contact lens materials. Int. Contact Lens Clin. 16:48–58.

Ang JHB, Efron N (1990): Corneal hypoxia and hypercapnia during contact lens wear. Optom. Vis. Sci 67:512–521.

Araie M, Maurice DM (1987): The rate of diffusion of fluorophores through the corneal epithelium and stroma. Exp. Eye Res. 44:73–87.

Ashton N (1951): Anatomical study of Schlemm's canal and aqueous veins by means of neoprene casts. Br. J. Ophthalmol. 35:291–303.

Barany EH (1959): On the mechanism by which chamber depth affects outflow resistance in excised eyes. Doc. Ophthalmol. 13:84–89.

Barany EH, Kinsey VE (1949): The rate of flow of aqueous humor. Am. J. Ophthalmol. 32(Pt. II):177–188.

Barr RE, Silver IA (1973): Effects of corneal environment on oxygen tension in the anterior chamber of rabbit. Invest. Ophthalmol. 12:140–144.

Battaglioli JL, Kamm RD (1984): Measurements of the compressive properties of scleral tissue. Invest. Ophthalmol. Vis. Sci. 25:59–65.

Baurmann M (1925): Über der Enstehung und klinische Bedeutung des Netzhautvenenpulses. Bericht deutsch Ophthalmologie Gesellschaft 45:53.

Becker B (1958): The decline in aqueous secretion and outflow facility with age. Am. J. Ophthalmol. 46:731–736.

Beems EM, Van Best JA (1990): Light transmission of the cornea in whole human eyes. Exp. Eye Res. 50(4):393–395.

Bergmanson JPG (1990): Clinical anatomy of the external eye. J. Am. Optom. Assoc. 61(Suppl. 6):S7–S15.

Bert JL, Fatt I (1969): Effect of convective flow on the oxygen tension profile in the cornea. Bull. Math. Biophys. 31:569–574.

Bert JL, Fatt I (1970): Relation of water transport to water content in swelling membranes. In Blank M (ed): Surface Chemistry of Biological Systems. New York, Plenum Press.

Berta A, Török M (1986): Soluble glycoproteins in aqueous tears. In Holly FJ (ed): The Preocular Tear Film in Health, Disease, and Contact Lens Wear, p. 506. Lubbock, TX, Dry Eye Institute.

Best M, Pola R, Galin MA, Blumenthal M (1970): Tonometric calibration for the rabbit eye. Arch. Ophthalmol. 84:200–205.

Bettelheim FA, Ali S (1985): Light scattering of normal human lens. III. Relationship between forward and back scatter of whole excised lenses. Exp. Eye Res. 41:1–9.

Bettelheim FA, Chylack LT (1985): Light scattering of whole excised human cataractous lenses. Relationships between different light scattering parameters. Exp. Eye Res. 41:19–30.

Bettelheim FA, Goetz D (1976): Distribution of hexosamines in bovine cornea. Invest. Ophthalmol. Vis. Sci. 15:301–304.

Bill A (1964): The drainage of albumin from the uvea. Exp. Eye Res. 3:179–187.

Bill A (1975): Blood circulation and fluid dynamics in the eye. Physiol. Rev. 55:383.

Bill A, Barany EH (1966): Gross facility, facility of conventional routes, and pseudofacility of aqueous humor outflow in the cynomolgus monkey. Arch. Ophthalmol. 75:665–673.

Bonanno JA, Polse KA (1987): Corneal acidosis during contact lens wear: effects of hypoxia and CO_2. Invest. Ophthalmol. Vis. Sci. 28:522–530.

Brencher HL, Kohl P, Reinke AR, Yolton RL (1991): Clinical comparison of air-puff and Goldmann tonometers. J. Am. Optom. Assoc. 62:395–402.

Brown M, Chinn S, Fatt I, Harris MG (1973): The effect of soft and hard contact lenses on blink rate, amplitude, and length. J. Am. Optom. Assoc. 44:254–257.

Brown SI, Dervichian DG (1969): The oils of the Meibomian glands. Arch. Ophthalmol. 82:537–540.

Brubaker RF, Riley FC Jr (1972): Vitreous body volume reduction in the rabbit. Arch. Ophthalmol. 87:438.

Cantrill HL, Pederson JE (1984): Experimental retinal detachment. VI. The permeability of the blood-retina barrier. Arch. Ophthalmol. 102:747–751.

Carney LG, Jacobs RF (1984): Mechanisms of visual loss in corneal edema. Arch. Ophthalmol. 102:1068–1071.

Carslaw HS, Jaeger J (1959): Conduction of Heat in Solids. Oxford, Oxford Press.

Carter DB (1972): Use of red blood cells to observe tear flow under contact lenses. Am. J. Optom. 49:617–618.

Castoro JA, Bettelheim AA, Bettelheim FA (1988): Water gradients across bovine cornea. Invest. Ophthalmol. Vis. Sci. 29:963–968.

Cohen AI (1975): The retina and optic nerve. In Moses RA (ed): Adler's Physiology of the Eye, 6th ed. St. Louis, CV Mosby.

Cohen LH, Noell WK (1960): Glucose catabolism of the rabbit retina before and after development of visual function. J. Neurochem. 5:253.

Cohen LH, Noell WK (1965): Relationship between visual function and metabolism. In Graymore CN (ed): Biochemistry of the Retina. New York, Academic Press.

Cole DF (1966): Aqueous humor formation. Doc. Ophthalmol. 21:116–238.

Costagliola C, Trapanese A, Pagano M (1990): Intraocular pressure in a healthy population: a survey of 751 subjects. Optom. Vis. Sci. 67(3):204–206.

Cox JL, Farrell RA, Hart RW, Langham ME (1970): The transparency of the mammalian cornea. J. Physiol. 210:601–616.

Cuklanz HD, Hill RM (1968): Tear space volumes of spherical and toric cornea-contact lens systems. Am. J. Optom. 45:719–734.

Cuklanz HD, Hill RM (1969): Oxygen requirements of corneal contact lens systems. Am. J. Optom. 46:228–230.

Daubs J (1976): A retrospective analysis of the systolic BP/IOP ratio in glaucoma screening. J. Am. Optom. Assoc. 47:450–455.

Davson H (1955): The hydration of the cornea. Biochem. J. 59:24.

Davson H (1956): Physiology of the Ocular and Cerebrospinal Fluids. Boston, Little, Brown.

Davson H (1962): The Eye, Vol 1. New York, Academic Press.

Davson H (ed) (1969): The Eye, Vol. 1, 2nd ed. New York, Academic Press.

Davson H, Spaziani E (1960): The fate of substances injected into the anterior chamber of the eye. J. Physiol. 151:202.

deGuillebon H, Zauberman H (1972): Experimental retinal detachment: biophysical aspects of retinal peeling and stretching. Arch. Ophthalmol. 87:545–548.

de Roetth A (1950): Respiration of the cornea. Arch. Ophthalmol. 44:666–676.

Doane MG (1980): Interaction of eyelids and tears in corneal wetting and the dynamics of the normal human eyeblink. Am. J. Ophthalmol. 89:507–516.

Doane MG, Gleason WJ (1991): Tear layer mechanisms. In Bennett ES, Weissman BA (eds): Clinical Contact Lens Practice, pp. 1–17. Philadelphia, JB Lippincott.

Dohlman CH (1971): The function of the epithelium in health and disease. Invest. Ophthalmol. Vis. Sci. 10(6):383–407.

Draeger J (1959): Untersuchungen über den Rigiditâlskoeffizienten. Doc. Ophthalmol. 13:431–486.

Drews RC (1971): Manual of Tonography. St. Louis, CV Mosby.

Duke-Elder S (1930): The nature of the vitreous body. Br. J. Ophthalmol. Mono., Suppl. 4:1–72.

Duke-Elder S (1968): System of Ophthalmology, Vol. IV: The Physiology of the Eye and of Vision. St. Louis, CV Mosby.

Duke-Elder S, Scott GI (1971): Neuro-ophthalmology. In Duke-Elder S (ed): System of Ophthalmology, Vol. 12, p. 893. London, Henry Kimpton.

Efron N, Carney LG (1979): Oxygen levels beneath the closed eyelid. Invest. Ophthalmol. Vis. Sci. 18:93–95.

Ehlers N (1966): The fibrillary texture and the hydration of the cornea. Acta Ophthalmol. 44:620–630.

Emsley HH (1963): Visual Optics, Vol. 1: Optics of Vision, 5th ed. London, Hatton Press.

Endo EG, Yao X-Y, Marmor MF (1988): Pigment adherence as a measure of retinal adhesion: dependence on temperature. Invest. Ophthalmol. Vis. Sci. 29:1390–1396.

Ericson LA (1958): Twenty-four hourly variations of the aqueous flow. Examination with perilimbal suction cup. Acta Ophthalmol. 36:381–385.

Fain GL, Matthews HR (1990): Calcium and the mechanism of light adaptation in vertebrate photoreceptors. Trends Neurosci. 13:378–384.

Farris RL, Takahashi GH, Donn A (1965): Oxygen flux across the in vivo rabbit cornea. Arch. Ophthalmol. 74(5):679–682.

Fatt I (1968a): Dynamics of water transport in the corneal stroma. Exp. Eye Res. 7:402–412.

Fatt I (1968b): Steady state distribution of oxygen and carbon dioxide in the in vivo cornea. II. The open eye in nitrogen and the covered eye. Exp. Eye Res. 7:413–430.

Fatt I (1969a): Permeability of Descemet's membrane to water. Exp. Eye Res. 8:340–354.

Fatt I (1969b): Oxygen tension under a contact lens during blinking. Am. J. Optom. 46:654–661.

Fatt I (1971a): The coefficient of thermal expansion of stroma. Exp. Eye Res. 12:254–260.

Fatt I (1971b): Influence of a hyperbaric environment on oxygen tension under a contact lens. Am. J. Optom. 48:109–112.

Fatt I (1975): Flow and diffusion in the vitreous body of the eye. Bull. Math. Biol. 37:85–90.

Fatt I (1976): The Polarographic Oxygen Sensor. Cleveland, CRC Press.

Fatt I (1977a): Hydraulic flow conductivity of the vitreous gel. Invest. Ophthalmol. 16:565–568.

Fatt I (1977b): A rational method for the design of gas-permeable soft contact lenses. The Optician (London) 173(4470):10–15.

Fatt I (1991): Observations of tear film break up on model eyes. CLAO J. 17:1–15.

Fatt I, Bieber MT (1968): The steady state distribution of oxygen and carbon dioxide in the in vivo cornea. I. The open eye in air and the closed eye. Exp. Eye Res. 7:103–112.

Fatt I, Bieber MT, Pye SD (1969): Steady state distribution of oxygen and carbon dioxide in the in vivo cornea of the eye covered by a gas-permeable contact lens. Am. J. Optom. 46:3–14.

Fatt I, Fink SE (1989): The ratio of carbon dioxide to oxygen permeability of RGP contact lens materials. Int. Contact Lens Clin. 11 and 12:347–352.

Fatt I, Freeman RD, Lin D (1974): Oxygen tension distributions in the cornea. A re-examination. Exp. Eye Res. 18:357–365.

Fatt I, Harris MG (1973): Refractive index of the cornea as a function of its thickness. Am. J. Optom. 50:383–386.

Fatt I, Hedbys BO (1970a): Flow conductivity of human corneal stroma. Exp. Eye Res. 10:237–242.

Fatt I, Hedbys BO (1970b): Flow of water in the sclera. Exp. Eye Res. 10:243–249.

Fatt I, Hill RM (1970): Oxygen tension under a contact lens during blinking—a comparison of theory and experimental observation. Am. J. Optom. 47:50–55.

Fatt I, Lin D (1976): Oxygen tension under a soft or hard gas-permeable contact lens in the presence of tear pumping. Am. J. Optom. Physiol. Opt. 53:104–111.

Fatt I, Liu SK-M (1984): Oxygen tension under a gas permeable hard contact lens. Int. Cont. Lens Clin. 11:93–105.

Fatt I, Hill RM, Takahashi GH (1964): Carbon dioxide efflux from the human cornea in vivo. Nature 203:738–740.

Fatt I, St Helen R (1971): Oxygen tension under an oxygen-permeable contact lens. Am. J. Optom. 48:545–555.

Fatt I, Shantinath K (1971): Flow conductivity of retina and its role in retinal adhesion. Exp. Eye Res. 12:218–226.

Fels IG (1970): Permeability of the anterior bovine lens capsule. Exp. Eye Res. 10:8–14.

Feuk T, McQueen D (1971): The angular dependence of light scattered from the rabbit cornea. Invest. Ophthalmol. Vis. Sci. 10:294–299.

Firberg TR, Lace JW (1988): A comparison of the elastic properties of human choroid and sclera. Exp. Eye Res. 47:429–436.

Forbes M, Pico G, Grolman B (1974): A noncontact applanation tonometer. Arch. Ophthalmol. 91:134–140.

Fowlks WL, Havener VR, Good JS (1963): Meridional flow from the corona ciliaris through the pararetinal zone of the rabbit vitreous. Invest. Ophthalmol. 2:63–71.

Frambach DA, Marmor MF (1982): The rate and route of fluid resorption from the subretinal space of the rabbit. Invest. Ophthalmol. Vis. Sci. 22:292–302.

Freddo TF, Bartels SP, Barsotti MF, Kamm RD (1990): The source of proteins in the aqueous humor of the normal rabbit. Invest. Ophthalmol. Vis. Sci. 31(1):125–137.

Freeman RD (1972): Oxygen consumption by the component layers of the cornea. J. Physiol. 225:15–32.

Freeman RD, Fatt I (1972): Oxygen permeability of the limiting layers of the cornea. Biophys. J. 12:237–247.

Freeman RD, Fatt I (1973): Environmental influences on ocular temperature. Invest. Ophthalmol. 12:596–602.

Friberg TR, Lace JW (1988): A comparison of the elastic properties of human choroid and sclera. Exp. Eye Res. 47:429–436.

Friedenwald JS (1937): Contributions to the theory and practice of tonometry. Am. J. Ophthalmol. 20:985–1024.

Friedenwald JS (1957): Tonometer calibration. An attempt to remove discrepancies found in the 1954 calibration scale for Schiøtz tonometers. Trans. Am. Acad. Ophthalmol. Otolaryngol. 61:108–123.

Gamm E (1980): The dependence of acid-base balance in the aqueous humor on carbon dioxide and oxygen diffusion through the cornea. Albrecht von Graefes Arch. Klin. Ophthalmol. 214:101–105.

Gloster J (1965): Tonometry and Tonography, Vol. 5, No. 4. International Ophthalmology Clinics. Boston, Little, Brown.

Goldmann H (1950): Über Fluorescein in der menschlichen Vorderkammer. Ophthalmologica 119:65–95.

Goldmann H, Schmidt T (1957): Über Applanations-Tonometrie. Ophthalmologica 134:221–242.

Gordon G (1951): Observations upon the movements of the eyelids. Br. J. Ophthalmol. 35:339–351.

Graham P, Hollows FC (1964): Sources of variation in tonometry. Trans. Ophthalmol. Soc. 84:597–613.

Graymore CN (1969): General aspects of the metabolism of the retina. In Davson H (ed): The Eye, Vol. 1: Vegetative Physiology and Biochemistry. New York, Academic Press.

Green K, Pedersen JE (1972): Contribution of secretion and filtration to aqueous humor formation. Am. J. Physiol. 222:1218.

Grolman B (1972): A new tonometer system. Am. J. Optom. 49:646–660.

Haberich FJ (1966): Quelques aspects physiologiques de l'adaption des verres de contact. Cahiers Verres Cont. 11:1–6.

Hale PN, Maurice DM (1969): Sugar transport across the corneal endothelium. Exp. Eye Res. 8:205–215.

Hamano H, Hori M, Hamano T, Kawabe H, Mikami M, Mitsuanaga S, Hamano T (1983): Effects of contact lens wear on mitosis of corneal epithelium and lactate content in aqueous humor of rabbit. Jpn J. Ophthalmol. 27:451–458.

Hara T, Maurice DM (1969): Epithelial damage and endothelial function in the cornea. Exp. Eye Res. 8:397–400.

Hara T, Maurice DM (1972): Changes in the swelling pressure of the corneal stroma with time, hydration and temperature, determined by a new method. Exp. Eye Res. 14:40–48.

Hart RW, Farrell RA (1969): Light scattering in the cornea. J. Opt. Soc. Am. 59:766–774.

Hayashi TT (1977): Mechanics of contact lens motion. Ph.D. Thesis. University of California, Berkeley.

Hayreh SS (1966): Posterior drainage of the intraocular fluid from the vitreous. Exp. Eye Res. 5:123.

Heald K, Langham ME (1956): Permeability of the cornea and the blood-aqueous barrier to oxygen. Br. J. Ophthalmol. 40(12):705–720.

Hedbys BO, Dohlman CH (1963): A new method for the determination of the swelling pressure of the corneal stroma in vitro. Exp. Eye Res. 2:122.

Hedbys BO, Mishima S (1962): Flow of water in the corneal stroma. Exp. Eye Res. 1:262.

Hedbys BO, Mishima S (1966): The thickness-hydration relationship of the cornea. Exp. Eye Res. 5:221–228.

Hedbys BO, Mishima S, Maurice DM (1963): The imbibition pressure of the corneal stroma. Exp. Eye Res. 2:99.

Henson DB (1983): Optometric Instruction, Chapter 3. London, Butterworths.

Hill RM, Fatt I (1963a): How dependent is the cornea on the atmosphere? J. Am. Optom. Assoc. 35:873–875.

Hill RM, Fatt I (1963b): Oxygen uptake from a reservoir of limited volume by the human cornea in vivo. Science 142:1295–1297.

Hill RM, Fatt I (1964): Oxygen measurements under a contact lens. Am. J. Optom. 41:382–387.

Hodson S (1977): The endothelial pump of the cornea. Invest. Ophthalmol. Vis. Sci. 16:589–591.

Hodson S, Miller F (1976): The bicarbonate ion pump in the endothelium which regulates the hydration of the rabbit cornea. J. Physiol. 263:563–577.

Hogan MJ, Alvarado JA, Weddell JE (1971): Histology of the Human Eye. Philadelphia, WB Saunders.

Holden BA, Mertz GW (1984): Critical oxygen levels to avoid corneal edema for daily and extended wear contact lenses. Invest. Ophthalmol. Vis. Sci. 25:1161–1167.

Holden BA, Sweeney DF, Sanderson G (1984): The minimal precorneal oxygen tension to avoid corneal edema. Invest. Ophthalmol. Vis. Sci. 25:450–476.

Holden BA, Sweeney DF, Vannas A (1985): Effects of long-term extended contact lens wear on the human cornea. Invest. Ophthalmol. Vis. Sci. 26:1489–1501.

Holden BA, Williams L, Zantos SG (1985): The etiology of transient endothelial changes in the human cornea. Invest. Ophthalmol. Vis. Sci. 10:1354–1359.

Holly FJ (1973): Formation and stability of the tear film. In Holly FJ, Lemp MA (eds): The Preocular Tear Film and Dry Eye Syndromes, Vol. 13, No. 1. International Ophthalmology Clinics. Boston, Little, Brown.

Hughes BA, Miller SS, Machen TE (1984): Effects of cyclic AMP on fluid absorption and ion transport across frog retinal pigment epithelium: measurements in the open-circuit state. J. Gen. Physiol. 83:875–899.

Isenberg SJ, Green BF (1985): Changes in conjunctival oxygen tension and temperature with advancing age. Crit. Care Med. 13:683–685.

Iwata S (1973): Chemical composition of the aqueous phase. In Holly FJ, Lemp MA (eds): The Preocular Tear Film and Dry Eye Syndromes. International Ophthalmology Clinics. Boston, Little, Brown.

Jacobi KW (1968): Sauerstoff Partialdruck messengen im Kammerwasser bei bedeutung mit verschiedenen Gasgermischen. Albrecht von Graefes Arch. Ophthalmol. 2174(4):321–325.

Jauregui M, Fatt I (1971): Estimation of oxygen tension under a contact lens. Am. J. Optom. 48:210–218.

Jauregui M, Fatt I (1972): Estimation of the in vivo oxygen consumption rate of the human corneal epithelium. Am. J. Optom. 49:507–511.

Jones RF, Maurice DM (1966): New methods of measuring the rate of aqueous flow in man with fluorescein. Exp. Eye Res. 5:208–220.

Kangas TA, Edelhauser HF, Twining SS, O'Brien WJ (1988): Loss of stromal proteoglycans during corneal edema. Invest. Ophthalmol. Vis. Sci. 29(Suppl.):215.

Kao SF, Lichter PR, Bergstrom TJ, Rowe S, Musch DC (1987): Clinical comparison of the ocular Tono-Pen to the Goldmann applanation tonometer. Ophthalmology 94:1541–1544.

Kapetansky FM, Higbee JW (1969): Vitreous deturgescense. Eye Ear Nose Throat Monthly 48:313.

Katchalsky A, Curran PF (1967): Nonequilibrium Thermodynamics in Biophysics. Cambridge, Harvard University Press.

Keeley FW, Morin JD, Vesely S (1984): Characterization of collagen from normal human sclera. Exp. Eye Res. 39:533–542.

Khan JA, LaGreca BA (1989): Tono-pen estimation of intraocular pressure through bandage contact lenses. Am. J. Ophthalmol. 108:422–425.

Kikkawa Y (1960): Light scattering studies of the rabbit cornea. Jap. J. Physiol. 10:292–302.

Kikkawa Y, Hirayama K (1970): Uneven swelling of the corneal stroma. Invest. Ophthalmol. Vis. Sci. 9:735–741.

Kinoshita JH, Masurat T, Helfant M (1955): Pathways of glucose metabolism in corneal epithelium. Science 122:72–73.

Kinsey VE (1947): Transfer of ascorbic acid and related compounds across the blood-aqueous barrier. Am. J. Ophthalmol. 30:1262–1266.

Kita M, Negi A, Kawano S, Honda Y, Maegawa S (1990): Measurement of retinal adhesive force in the in vivo rabbit eye. Invest. Ophthalmol. Vis. Sci. 31:624–628.

Kitazawa Y, Horie T (1975): Diurnal variation of intraocular pressure in primary open angle glaucoma. Am. J. Ophthalmol. 79:557–566.

Kleinstein RN, Fatt I (1977): Pressure dependency of trans-scleral flow. Exp. Eye Res. 24:335–340.

Kleinstein RM, Kwan M, Fatt I, Weissman BA (1981): In vivo aqueous humor oxygen tension—as estimated from measurements on bare stroma. Invest. Ophthalmol. Vis. Sci. 21(3):415–421.

Klyce SD (1981): Stromal lactate accumulation can account for corneal edema osmotically following epithelial hypoxia in the rabbit. J. Physiol. 321:49–64.

Klyce SD, Crosson CE (1985): Transport processes across the corneal epithelium: a review. Curr. Eye Res. 4:323–331.

Klyce S, Dohlman CH, Tolpin DW (1971): In vivo determination of corneal swelling pressure. Exp. Eye Res. 11:220.

Kolker AE, Hetherington J (1983): Becker-Shaffer's diagnosis and therapy of the glaucomas, ed. 3. St. Louis, CV Mosby.

Koretz, JF, Handelman GH (1988): How the human eye focuses. Sci. Am. 259(1):92–99.

Kruse W (1960): Eine neue Messmethode des Rigiditatskoeffizienten. Albrecht von Graefes Arch. Ophthalmol. 162:78–96.

Kuck JFR Jr (1961): The formation of fructose in the ocular lens. AMA Arch. Ophthalmol. 65:840–846.

Kuwabara T, Cogan DG (1961): Retinal glycogen. Arch. Ophthalmol. 66:680–688.

Kwan M, Fatt I (1970): A noninvasive method of continuous arterial oxygen tension estimation from measured palpebral conjunctival oxygen tension. Anesthesiology 35:309.

Lambert SR, Klyce SD (1981): The origins of Sattler's veil. Am. J. Ophthalmol. 91:51–56.

Larke JR, Parrish ST, Wigham CG (1981): Apparent human corneal oxygen uptake rate. Am. J. Optom. Physiol. Opt. 58(10):803–805.

Lerman S (1984): Biophysical aspects of corneal and lenticular transparency. Curr. Eye Res. 3(1):3–13.

Leydhecker W, Akiyama K, Newmann HG (1958): Der intraokulare Druck gesunder menschlicher Augen. Klin. Monatsbl. Augenheilkd. 133:662.

Linnér E (1958): Changeability test of aqueous outflow resistance. Br. J. Ophthalmol. 42:38–53.

Linsenmeier RA, Goldstick TK, Blum RS, Enroth-Cugell C (1981): Estimation of retinal oxygen transients from measurements made into the vitreous humor. Exp. Eye Res. 32:369–379.

Linsenmeier RA, Yancey CM (1989): Effects of hyperoxia on the oxygen distribution in the intact cat retina. Invest. Ophthalmol. Vis. Sci. 30:612–618.

Mandell RB, Farrell R (1980): Corneal swelling at low atmospheric oxygen pressures. Invest. Ophthalmol. Vis. Sci. 19:697–702.

Mandell RB, Fatt I (1965): Thinning of the human cornea on awakening. Nature 208:292–293.

Mandell RB, Harris MG (1968): Theory of the contact lens adaptation process. J. Am. Optom. Assoc. 39:260–261.

Marmor MF, Abdul-Rahim AS, Cohen DS (1980): The effect of metabolic inhibitors on retinal adhesion and subretinal fluid resorption. Invest. Ophthalmol. Vis. Sci. 19:893.

Masters BR (1984): Oxygen tensions of rabbit corneal epithelium measured by non-invasive redox fluorometry. Invest. Ophthalmol. Vis. Sci (ARVO Abstracts) 25 (Suppl.):102.

Maurice DM (1951): The permeability to sodium ions of the living rabbit's cornea. J. Physiol. 122:367–391.

Maurice DM (1955): Influence on corneal permeability of bathing with solutions of differing reaction and tonicity. Br. J. Ophthalmol. 39:463–473.

Maurice DM (1957a): The exchange of sodium between the vitreous body and the blood and aqueous humor. J. Physiol. 137:110–125.

Maurice DM (1957b): The structure and transparency of the cornea. J. Physiol. 136:263–286.

Maurice DM (1959): Protein dynamics in the eye studied with labelled proteins. Am. J. Ophthalmol. 47(Pt. 2):361–368.

Maurice DM (1967): The use of fluorescein in ophthalmological research. Invest. Ophthalmol. 6:464–477.

Maurice DM (1969): The cornea and the sclera. In Davson H (ed): The Eye, Vol. 1. New York, Academic Press.

Maurice DM (1972): The location of the fluid pump in the cornea. J. Physiol. 221:43–54.

Maurice DM (1984): The cornea and sclera. In Davson H (ed): The Eye, 3rd ed. Orlando, Academic Press.

Maurice DM, Giardini AA (1951): Swelling of the cornea in vivo after the destruction of its limiting layers. Br. J. Ophthalmol. 35:791–797.

Maurice DM, Monroe F (1990): Cohesive strength of corneal lamellae. Exp. Eye Res. 50(1):59–63.

Maurice DM, Polgar J (1977): Diffusion across the sclera. Exp. Eye Res. 25:577–582.

Maurice DM, Riley MV (1968): The biochemistry of the cornea. In Graymore CN (ed): The Biochemistry of the Eye. New York, Academic Press.

Maurice DM, Salmon J, Zauberman H (1971): Subretinal pressure and retinal adhesion. Exp. Eye Res. 12:212–217.

Maurice DM, Watson PG (1965): The distribution and movement of serum albumin in the cornea. Exp. Eye Res. 4:355–363.

McDonagh AF, Nguyen ML (1989): Spectacles, ultraviolet radiation, and formation of cataracts. N. Engl. J. Med. 321:1478–1479.

McDonald JE, Brubaker S (1971): Meniscus-induced thinning of tear films. Am. J. Ophthalmol. 72:139–146.

McEwen WK, St. Helen R (1965): Rheology of the human sclera. Ophthalmologica 150:321–346.

McLeod SD, West SK, Quigley HA, Fozzard JL (1990): A longitudinal study of the relationship between intraocular and blood pressure. Invest. Ophthal. Vis. Sci. 31:2361–2366.

McMillan F, Forster RK (1975): Comparison of Mackay-Marg, Goldmann and Perkins tonometers in abnormal corneas. Arch. Ophthalmol. 93:420–424.

Merriam FC, Kinsey VE (1950): Studies on the crystalline lens. II. Incorporation of glycine and serine in the protein of lenses cultured in vitro. Arch. Ophthalmol. 44:651–658.

Michels RG, Wilkenson CP, Rice TA (1990): Retinal Detachment. St. Louis, CV Mosby.

Miller SS, Hughes BA, Machen TE (1982): Fluid transport across retinal pigment epithelium is inhibited by cyclic AMP. Proc. Natl. Acad. Sci. USA 79:2111.

Millidot M, O'Leary DJ (1980): Effect of oxygen deprivation on corneal sensitivity. Acta Ophthalmol. 58:434–439.

Mishima S, Hedbys BO (1967): The permeability of the corneal epithelium and endothelium to water. Exp. Eye Res. 6:10–32.

Mishima S, Maurice DM (1961a): The effect of normal evaporation on the eye. Exp. Eye Res. 1:46–52.

Mishima S, Maurice DM (1961b): The oily layer of the tear film and evaporation from the corneal surface. Exp. Eye Res. 1:39–45.

Molnar I, Poitry S, Tsacopoulos M, Gilodi N, Leuenberger PM (1985): Effect of laser photocoagulation on oxygenation of the retina in miniature pigs. Invest. Ophthalmol. Vis. Sci. 26:1410–1414.

Mondino BJ, Brady KF (1981): Distribution of hemolytic complement in the normal cornea. Arch. Ophthalmol. 99:1430–1433.

Mondino BJ, Sundar-Raj CV, Brady KJ (1982): Production of first component of complement by corneal fibroblasts in tissue culture. Arch. Ophthalmol. 100:478–480.

Negi A, Marmor MF (1986): Quantitative estimation of metabolic transport of subretinal fluid. Invest. Ophthalmol. Vis. Sci. 27:1564–1568.

Norn MS (1969): Desiccation of the precorneal film. I. Corneal wetting time. Acta Ophthalmol. 47:865–870.

Novack RL, Stefansson E, Hatchell DL (1990): The effect of photocoagulation on the oxygenation and ultrastructure of avascular retina. Exp. Eye Res. 50:289–296.

O'Leary DJ, Wilson G, Henson DB (1981): The effect of anoxia on the human corneal epithelium. Am. J. Optom. Physiol. Opt. 58:472–476.

O'Neal MR, Polse KA, Sarver MD (1984): Corneal response to rigid and hydrogel lenses during eye closure. Invest. Ophthalmol. Vis. Sci. 25:837–842.

Ota Y, Mishima S, Maurice DM (1974): Endothelial permeability of the living cornea to fluorescein. Invest. Ophthalmol. Vis. Sci. 13(12):945–949.

Payrau P, Pouliquen Y, Faure J-P, Offret G (1967): La Transparence de la Cornée. Paris, Masson et Cie.

Pedersen JE, Green K (1973): Aqueous humor dynamics: experimental studies. Exp. Eye Res. 15:277–297.

Pirie A (1969): The vitreous body. In Davson H (ed): The Eye, Vol. 1. New York, Academic Press.

Pitts DG, Bergmanson JPG, Chu LWF (1987): Ultrastructural analysis of corneal exposure to UV radiation. Acta Ophthalmol. 65:263–273.

Polse KA, Mandell RB (1970): Critical oxygen tension at the corneal surface. Arch. Ophthalmol. 84:505–508.

Polse KA, Mandell RB (1971): Hyperbaric oxygen effect on corneal edema caused by a contact lens. Am. J. Optom. 48:197–200.

Port MJA, Asaria TS (1990): The assessment of human tear volume. J. Br. Contact Lens Assoc. 13:76–82.

Pournaras CJ, Riva CE, Tsacopoulos M, Strommer K (1989): Diffusion of O_2 in the retina of anesthetized miniature pigs in normoxia and hyperoxia. Exp. Eye Res. 49:347–360.

Prijot E (1961): Contribution à l'étude de la tonometrie. Doc. Ophthalmol. 15:7–225.

Prince JH (1964): The Rabbit in Eye Research. Springfield, IL, Charles C Thomas.

Riley MV (1969): Glucose and oxygen utilization by the rabbit cornea. Exp. Eye Res. 8:193–200.

Riley MV (1977): A study of the transfer of amino acids across the endothelium of the rabbit cornea. Exp. Eye Res. 24:35–44.

Robbins R, Galin MA (1969): Effect of osmotic agents on the vitreous body. Arch. Ophthalmol. 82:694–699.

Rohen JW (1979): Scanning electron microscopic studies of the zonular apparatus in human and monkey eyes. Invest. Ophthalmol. Vis. Sci. 18(2):133–144.

Ross EJ (1951): The transfer of non-electrolytes across the blood-aqueous barrier. J. Physiol. 112:229–237.

Ross EJ (1952): The influence of insulin on the permeability of the blood aqueous barrier to glucose. J. Physiol. 116:414–423.

Saeteren T (1960): Further investigations of aqueous flow in normal eyes after compression. Acta Ophthalmol. 38:496–523.

Schoessler JP (1987): Contact lens wear and the corneal endothelium. J. Am. Optom. Assoc. 58(10):804–810.

Sears ML (1981): The aqueous. In Moses RA (ed): Adler's Physiology of the Eye. St. Louis, CV Mosby.

Smelser GK, Ozanics V (1952): Importance of atmospheric oxygen for maintenance of the optical properties of the human cornea. Science 115:140.

Sorensen PN (1975): The noncontact tonometer. Clinical evaluation on normal and diseased eyes. Acta Ophthalmol. 53:513–521.

Spector A (1984): The search for a solution to senile cataracts. Invest. Ophthalmol. Vis. Sci. 25(2):130–146.

Stanley JA (1972): Water permeability of the human cornea. Arch. Ophthalmol. 87:568–573.

Stefansson E, Wolbarsht ML, Landers MB (1983): In vivo O_2 consumption in rhesus monkeys in light and dark. Exp. Eye Res. 37:251–256.

Swann HG (1954): The physiologic constructions in the ocular veins. Am. J. Ophthalmol. 38:845–850.

Thoft RA, Friend J (1971): Corneal epithelial glucose utilization. Arch. Ophthalmol. 88:58–62.

Tillis TN, Murray DL, Schmidt GJ, Weiter JJ (1988): Preretinal oxygen changes in the rabbit under conditions of light and dark. Invest. Ophthalmol. Vis. Sci. 29:988–991.

Trenberth SM, Mishima S (1968a): Permeability of the corneal endothelium to nonelectrolytes. Invest. Ophthalmol. Vis. Sci. 7:34–43.

Trenberth SM, Mishima S (1968b): The effect of ouabain on the rabbit corneal endothelium. Invest. Ophthalmol. 7:44–52.

Uniacke CA, Hill RM (1972): The depletion course of epithelial glycogen with corneal anoxia. Arch. Ophthalmol. 87(1):56–59.

Uniacke CA, Hill RM, Greenberg M, Seward S (1972): Physiological tests for new contact lens materials. Am. J. Optom. Arch. Am. Acad. Optom. 49:329–332.

Usukura J, Fain GL, Bok D (1988): [3H]Ouabain localization of Na-K ATPase in the epithelium of rabbit ciliary body pars plicata. Invest. Ophthalmol. Vis. Sci. 29(4):606–613.

van Heyningen R (1962): The sorbitol pathway in the lens. Exp. Eye Res. 1:396–404.

Verhagen C, Breeboart AC, Kijlsra A (1990): Diffusion of immunoglobin G from the vascular compartment into the normal rabbit cornea. Invest. Ophthalmol. Vis. Sci. 31(8):1519–1525.

Wagner L, Polse KA, Mandell RB (1980): Tear pumping and edema with soft contact lenses. Invest. Ophthalmol. Vis. Sci. 19:1397–1400.

Walls GL (1942): The Vertebrate Eye and Its Adaptive Radiation. Bloomfield, MI, Cranbrook Institute of Science (reprinted by Edwards Bros., Ann Arbor, MI).

Waring GO, Bourne WM, Edelhauser HF, Kenyon KR (1982): The corneal endothelium: normal and pathological structure and function. Ophthalmology 89:531–590.

Weekers R, Prijot E, Delmarcell Y, Lavergne G, Watillon M, Gouguard L, Gouguard-Rion C, Gustin J (1959): The early diagnosis of incipient glaucoma. Bull. Soc. Belge. Ophthalmol. 121:1.

Weissman BA, Blaze PA, Ingles S, Wheeler N (1988): Open-eye corneal swelling secondary to hydrogel contact lens wear. Am. J. Optom. Physiol. Opt. 65:272–276.

Weissman BA, Fatt I, Rasson J (1981): Diffusion of oxygen in human corneas in vivo. Invest. Ophthalmol. Vis. Sci. 20:123–125.

Weissman BA, Selzer K, Duffin RM, Pettit TH (1983): Oxygen permeability of rabbit and human corneal stroma. Invest. Ophthalmol. Vis. Sci. 24(5):645–647.

Wiig H (1989): Cornea fluid dynamics I: measurement of hydrostatic and colloid osmotic pressure in rabbits. Exp. Eye Res. 49:1015–1030.

Wiig H (1990): Corneal fluid dynamics. II. Evidence for transport of radiolabelled albumin in rabbits by bulk flow. Exp. Eye Res. 50:261–267.

Wilson GS, Fatt I (1974): Thickness changes in the epithelium of the excised rabbit cornea. Am. J. Optom. 51:75–83.

Wilson GS, Fatt I, Freeman RD (1973): Thickness changes in the stroma of an excised cornea during anoxia. Exp. Eye Res. 17:165–171.

Yancey CM, Linsenmeier RA (1989): Oxygen distribution and consumption in the cat retina at increased intraocular pressure. Invest. Ophthalmol. Vis. Sci. 30:600–611.

Yao X-Y, Endo EG, Marmor MF (1989): Reversibility of retinal adhesion in the rabbit. Invest. Ophthalmol Vis. Sci. 30:220–224.

Yee RW, Matsuda M, Schultz RO, Edelhauser HF (1985): Changes in the normal corneal endothelial cellular pattern as a function of age. Curr. Eye Res. 4:671–678.

Young RW (1967): The renewal of photoreceptor cell outer segments. J. Cell Biol. 33:61.

Ytteborg J, Dohlman CH (1965): Corneal edema and intraocular pressure. II. Clinical results. Arch. Ophthalmol. 74:477–484.

Yu DY, Cringle SJ, Adler VA (1990): The response of rat vitreal oxygen tension to stepwise increases in inspired percentage oxygen. Invest. Ophthalmol. Vis. Sci. 31:2193–2500.

Zauberman H, Berman ER (1969): Measurement of adhesive forces between the sensory retina and the pigment epithelium. Exp. Eye Res. 8:276–283.

Zauberman H, de Guillebon H (1972): Retinal traction in vivo and postmortem. Arch. Ophthalmol. 87:549–554.

Zucker BB (1966): Hydration and transparency of corneal stroma. Arch. Ophthalmol. 75:228–231.

Zuckerman R, Weiter JJ (1980): Oxygen transport in the bullfrog retina. Exp. Eye Res. 30:117–127.

Index

soluble protein content of, 80
solute transport in, 82–84
surface of, 11
water absorption of, 80
water content of, 77–78
Vitreous chamber, 2f, 11
Vitreous filtrate, 78
Vitreous gel, breakdown of, with age, 10
Vitreous humor, 78
Vitreous-retinal interface, 7
Vortex veins, 13

W
Water, bulk flow of, 118

Water-provocative test, for glaucoma, 76
Wing cells, 98–99, 100f, 101

X
Xpert noncontact tonometer(s), 55
Xylose, in aqueous humor, 22

Z
Zonulae occludens, 19
Zonule of Zinn, 9–10, 88, 88f
posterior leaf of, 11